- About the Author -

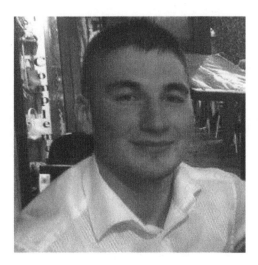

Scott Murray is a Health and Wellness advisor in the city of Aberdeen, Scotland/UK. He is qualified as a Level 3 Personal Trainer and started his own business in 2013 called 'Momentum Personal Development.' His job involves helping clients to reach their optimum health and fitness levels through consultations, exercise programmes and personal training sessions.

With time and experience he discovered his true passion lays in general health, physique and wellness for the average person looking to develop healthy habits and routines in their lives. This led him to pursue a career in writing about holistic health, and produce his first book 'Strip The Fat & Look Good In That.'

The book aims to serve as a practical blueprint covering all the key areas of health, including: exercise, nutrition, weight loss, cooking and recipes, supplements, positive life habits, mind-set, strategies, and exercise planning. As an author, he plans to write more books on other important areas relevant to human lifestyle such as: relationships, leadership, financial, success/life, and universal laws.

D1614876

Strip the Fat & Look Good in That

"Your Own Practical Blueprint for Natural Weight loss, Looking Lean, and Living a Positive, Healthy, and Vibrant Lifestyle"

Email: momentum-personal-development@hotmail.co.uk
Website: www.momentumupersonaldevelopment.co.uk

Strip the Fat & Look Good in That

Scott Murray

Akasha Publishing

Akasha Publishing Ltd
145-157 St John Street
London
England
EC1V 4PW

A CIP record for this book is available from the British library.

ISBN-13: 978-1-910246-07-8
ISBN-10: 1-910246-07-7

Printed and bound by Lightning Source

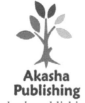

**Akasha
Publishing**
www.akashapublishing.co.uk
info@akashapublishing.co.uk

Acknowledgements

To everyone who has been there for me
and stayed close over the years, particularly
my close family and friends. Also to those
who have always believed I could do what
I set out to achieve.

- Contents -

- Introduction -

Y ou've been drawn to this book at this moment in time for a reason. I already know that you are looking for something new and different that you can apply in your life. If your goal is to lose weight, develop a more attractive physique and improve your health then this is the book for you.

You have already taken the first step towards a leaner, fitter, healthier you. There are more people today with major health problems attributed to unhealthy life styles than ever before. The old ways of doing things no longer produce the greatest results. In fact, the old ways have shaped much of how society now thinks and behaves, and are responsible for many of today's health problems.

In order to stay ahead and on top of *your own game*, it makes sense to upgrade your old ways of thinking and therefore your behaviour, for your overall wellbeing. Regardless of your current level of health or fitness, whether you're overweight, have a sedentary lifestyle or are a young, highly active athlete, by following the ideas and teachings presented in this book, you'll not only create positive and lasting changes in your outward physical appearance, but you will also be living your life from a much healthier, vibrant and higher energy state of health; not just today but every day for the rest of your life.

All you need to do is make the **decision** to change. I truly appreciate the time I am asking you to invest in reading and applying the principles and ideas presented in this book. I am certain that when you do; you will be amazed with the results. But why should you listen to me? Let me share part of my own journey and show you…

"If you don't like how things are, change it! You're not a tree."
– Jim Rohn

My Story

My passion was gone. I was standing in the gym looking at everyone around me diligently performing functional exercises, lifting weights or seated on fixed weight machines. Another personal trainer nearby was about to start a circuit class. And suddenly I knew it.
    I was done!
    I no longer had the same desire, meaning or belief in my work. The dream I had invested all my energies into for the past five years was over. Fitness and exercise have always been second nature to me, whether running around in the woods as a child or late night training sessions, punching away on a heavy bag in a private boxing gym. It has never been a chore, only a necessity. But something had changed and I knew it as I stood there in the gym that day.
    I ended my career as a personal trainer, just like that. I always believed it was my dream job; all that time and money I had invested travelling all over the country: education courses, long hours in classrooms designing exercise programs and lifting heavy tyres outdoors while mud and rain ran down my face.
    I'd read hundreds of books on health, nutrition and exercise, worked with no days off, hardly any social life and rarely saw my friends or family. And all for what? What would I do now?
    The excuse I had made for myself was *"I was burnt out"* – but it was easy to make excuses; to blame it on the long hours, when really it was something inside telling me there was another way. The break from my job gave me the time and distance I think I needed to really think about what I wanted next from my life.
    I started to miss my clients, but inside I felt a new kind of energy; new ideas beginning to form. Maybe I could still work in the same field, but find a different way; a way that would provide a more effective and powerful system for transforming the lives of my clients. I knew there had to be a reason for that moment, that day, in

the gym that made me stand back and re-examine my life and its purpose.

After spending some quiet time thinking and looking deep within myself, the answer came. What I really needed was a new challenge, something different that would stretch me both personally and professionally; something that would allow me to grow and develop as a person in the process. Instead of training fifteen to twenty regular clients at any one time, repeating the same routines day in and day out, I needed to leverage myself and my contribution in order be more effective and create a permanent and lasting impact on others.

So I decided I would write this book. I would redirect my passion into a single product that would reach far more people than my training could alone; a book that would empower others to also take charge of their lives and achieve the kind of transformations both physically and mentally that I know every one of you is capable of.

This book combines not only what I have learned about exercise and nutrition as a trainer, but provides a system that draws from psychology, science and the fundamental laws of the universe. It's a system that will enable you to change, but also to maintain that change – (forever).

My aim is to lift others to higher levels in their lives. So, to make that happen, I went back to work as a chef; my first profession, and worked hours that enabled my writing. Working from early in the morning until late afternoon, Monday to Friday, I was able to free up my evenings after boxing training to write.

I also worked as a club doorman during the weekends at a local nightclub to help fund the costs of living while I pursued the new dream.

"A journey of a thousand miles starts with a single step."
- Chinese Proverb

The Shape of Today

We are all hugely influenced by the media and by our community. Unconsciously we fall prey to negative ways of living and eating, and this puts us in the middle of a worldwide obesity epidemic. At no other time in history has such a high percentage of our population been so overweight. With it, come health problems like type 2 diabetes, cardiovascular disease and hypertension, all of which can be attributed to poor eating and lifestyle habits.

If left unchecked, these can easily progress into potentially fatal strokes and heart attacks. It's no surprise that we've got to this point. Every time we turn on the TV, advertisements glorify the worst possible foods; foods that are killing us slowly. Walk into any shop and you will be faced with shelves full of sugary sweets, drinks and highly processed, chemical-ridden foods.

Meanwhile, fresh grocery or butchers' stores are replaced by supermarkets with only a few aisles dedicated to foods that contain beneficial nutrients. Around our towns, count all the signs advertising fast food restaurants like McDonald's, Burger King and KFC. When was the last time you saw an advert selling fresh fruit and vegetables?

It is highly likely your family and friends enjoy a takeaway at the weekend. Gone are the days when the human race was lean, fit, strong and self-reliant. Many of us now struggle to carry the shopping to the car. We've gone from roaming the forests with a spear; fearless, strong and living in harmony with nature, to slouching over an office chair with a Coke and a Big Mac and fries.

The majority of us have become victims of our environment, developing bad postures and eating habits that result in large quantities of excess body fat. I will address many of the causes of this and then provide you with a new way of behaving. There is always a better path to choose.

So shake off self-limiting assumptions or beliefs, accumulated over the years from the people and environments around you, and make a choice right now to improve. If you choose to put into action the things in this book you will empower yourself and begin the process of change.

Don't blame your genetics, time constraints, work or the people around you. Some things may be harder for you to overcome, but by making small, reasonable progress, and by developing the habit of being fully responsible for yourself, you'll soon notice that you have outgrown all your unproductive ways of thinking and living.

And you'll have the people around you wondering what your big secret is. **So take responsibility**; focus on improvement by taking continual positive action. *Let the results that you're about to create, speak for themselves.*

"Don't wait. The time will never be just right."
– Napoleon Hill

What I Ask of You: Personal Investment

It's important for you to view this book as an **investment** in your future. This book is about something every human being should make a priority: **health.** Your body is all you have to live in and therefore your health is the foundation upon which all the other activities and areas of your life are built. Without health what are you?

Therefore your health truly deserves your greatest attention and not just from time to time but all throughout your life. I have never been ill or suffered from any illness or disease for as long as I can remember, going right back to early childhood. This is something I'm really proud of and I believe is possible for all of us simply by living your lives in a clean and active way.

By applying the system outlined in this book; by investing a few hours of exercise and thought to your nutritional needs, you will save yourself a lot of time, energy and money. Avoid the latest fads, the yo-yoing from periods of dieting and exercise and then periods without any. Change your thinking and invest in yourself – you'll be amazed at what can be achieved in a short space of time.

5

"If you are under the impression you have already perfected yourself, you will never rise to the heights you are no doubt capable of."
– Kazuo Ishiguro

The System

The system outlined in this book has been designed as a practical guide that you can begin to put into action right away.

Action must be your goal.

The information included is based on my professional education and grounded in science. Of course today there are many scientific studies and we can suffer from information overload. To add to the confusion, many findings are contradictory. This can be counterproductive, causing confusion and therefore inaction.

While scientific research may provide interesting reading, putting these findings into a positive action plan is not always easy or practical. So while I will draw upon solid science, my focus is to look at simple ways to create action from it and therefore produce permanent change.

What I can tell you are that all my methods and teachings come from what **"I know actually works"**; I've seen it for myself. That's why I'm sharing them with you and because I know we all have such busy lives, I am keeping it as *simple* as possible.

It's all about returning to the basics; eating higher quality foods, in smaller amounts, at the right times and incorporating regular physical activity. It's also about how we set our minds to maintain this. I won't pretend to have all the answers but I can assure you, and after many years of research, that what I am offering does produce quality **results.**

Just by following my system I can guarantee that you'll see changes occurring with each day. What better way to start your day than with a great feeling of control and contentment in your weight, physique and above all your health.

"Knowledge is power. It is nothing of the sort! Knowledge is only potential power. It becomes power only when, and if, it is organized into definite plans of action, and directed to a definite end."
— **Napoleon Hill**

The Starting Point is Desire

It's not enough for you to accept full personal responsibility and then make a clear decision to change. You have to want it – *really* want it. How much do *you* want it?

Desire is the fundamental motivation for action to truly succeed in anything. The desire to change must be fuelled by the positive outcomes you imagine for yourself and your health. It must be something you want deep inside and not the result of someone else's expectations or desires. Simply saying that you want to get great results is not enough. You must *truly desire* to become a better version of yourself, both physically and mentally, by making a few new efforts, repeated every day. If you don't possess a strong underlying desire to improve your current situation, you won't stick to it.

If you don't truly want to get rid of your excess weight and body fat, then you're not going to be able to keep your weight down for very long. If your desire isn't strong enough; if your inner values are not in alignment with your goals, then you are only going to let yourself down by reverting back to old habits.

Like most of us who make New Year resolutions, the results are short term, so you have to make a life change, and that means forever – not a short-term resolution you are going to break but a forever *no going back change*. And for that, you have to want it. Don't just do it for a loved one or even a doctor: **do it because you desire it above all else.**

You have to fully immerse yourself into this self-improvement process and to do that – it's all about you. The process of learning and putting your new levels of understanding into action should now be your focus.

"Don't judge yourself by your past; you no longer live there."
– Ifeanyi Enoch Onuoha

It Doesn't Matter Where You're Coming From all that Matters is Where You're Going. You can let the past, or failed attempts to create the new leaner, fitter, healthier you be the barrier to your success or you can finally let the past go.

Every moment in our lives we are dying and being born again into a new present moment. Nothing stays still. Everything is changing. Your past, no matter how great or how unfortunate it was, *is gone*. All you can do is cherish memories, forgive wrongs and realign your focus on what it is that you want most right now.

Take whatever lessons or wisdom you have gained from your past, into your present – so that you can put it to best use now and in your future. All you really have in your life is this moment. There will never be a right time in your life to learn and begin taking the positive actions to improve your health and physique so don't wait for one – **do it now.**

The chapters in this book will provide the most effective and powerful methods and actions that you can put to work in your life right now. The level of results and quality of health that you ultimately attain is completely dependent on you.

"Strive to be better today than you were yesterday better today than you were yesterday."
– James Gordon

Positive Changes

I don't believe in fate, I believe that we are in control of our own destiny. The universal law of Cause and Effect says **we get out, what we put in.** It's that simple.

Learning occurs best when we *want to learn*. To create lasting change, and improve ourselves, we must put all our learning *into action*. When we first begin we need willpower and discipline to take that first step but, after that, the results from those new productive habits will keep us going.

I will share with you some stories that show how strong wills have overcome incredible hardships. These are people who took full responsibility for their lives, no matter how difficult, proving that nothing is impossible unless you make it so.

1. Helen Keller

Helen Adams Keller was born June 27, 1880. At nineteen months Helen survived a terrible life-threatening fever which left her completely blind, deaf and unable to communicate. Helen's quality of life was extremely poor, living much like an animal, until the age of seven when her parents contacted a school for the blind in desperate need of help. That came in the form of Ann Sullivan. Ann worked tirelessly with Helen, teaching her letters, how to behave, how to talk and slowly allowed her to reconnect with the world.

Fuelled by her achievements, Helen developed an unrelenting desire to learn and soon learned how to read and write Braille. This opened up the world even more; enabling Helen to enrol in college, where she took classes alongside students who didn't share her challenges.

Consequently, she had to devote more time and attention to her studies than the average student. Helen eventually graduated from college, wrote and published her own book, learned five different languages and was the first blind-deaf person to ever receive a BA degree. Helen was a woman with a strong spirit of determination and persistence, showing that it doesn't matter if a person has a disability or a limitation because with hard work and faith one can still achieve anything.

Today Helen Keller is a role model and source of inspiration to many deaf and blind people around the world. She even founded an organisation that still helps to prevent blindness while teaching people how to live with their disabilities.

2. Oprah Winfrey

Oprah Winfrey spent the first six years of her life living with her grandmother in poverty, wearing dresses made from potato sacks. After being molested by two members of her family and a family friend, she ran away from home at thirteen.

At fourteen she gave birth to a baby who died shortly afterwards. She went back to live with her mother, who then sent her away to live with her father where she managed to turn her life around.

Oprah succeeded it attaining a full scholarship to college where she won a beauty pageant that lead to her being discovered by a radio station; the platform that launched her career and the many successes that followed. Today Oprah is a highly successful actress and has her own worldwide TV show where she has achieved billionaire status doing what she loves.

She is an inspiration to many, proving it doesn't matter where you came from; only where you're heading.

3. Thomas Edison

Thomas Edison is claimed to be one of the world's best inventors. While at school, Thomas's teachers said that he was "too stupid to learn anything" and he was fired from his first two jobs for being "non-productive". However Edison became an inventor by trade and after a thousand unsuccessful attempts he invented the light bulb and changed the face of history.

When a reporter asked him how it felt to fail a thousand times, Edison replied: "I didn't fail a thousand times. The light bulb was an invention of a thousand steps and I never quit."

View all set-backs as temporary. See every failure as a step closer to realising your dream.

"Anyone who stops learning is old, whether at twenty or eighty. Anyone who keeps learning stays young. The greatest thing in life is to keep your mind young."
– Henry Ford

-1-

Why Lose Weight and Get Healthy?

"It takes half your life before you discover life is a do-it-yourself project."
– **Napoleon Hill**

Two Paths, One Choice

No one else but you is responsible for how you look and how you feel. You are the one who decides what you eat and how much you exercise.

The universe is governed by hundreds of laws. Let's look more closely at the Law of Cause and Effect by giving you an example. Let's say you're engaged in moderate exercise five days a week, eat a few balanced, highly nutritious meals each day and repeat this pattern for two months, while avoiding foods high in fat and sugar. Good, right? Or you choose to hardly move from the couch every day for the same two months and eat fatty foods and sugar to excess.

Clearly the outcomes will be very different. Every action has a consequence. Does a stressful work situation cause you to sit in front of the TV with your hand dipped into a large bag of crisps, or does it put you in your gym clothes and see you working off those frustrations on a treadmill? **The way you act is a choice.** That choice is based on your beliefs, values and thought processes, whether you're conscious of it or not. Changes don't happen overnight and you can't make yourself thin overnight, but you can make the choice to change your life right now.

"It is our choices that show what we truly are far more than our abilities."
– J.K. Rowling

Law of Cause and Effect will help you change the following:

Physique:

1. Weight loss. Becoming a smaller version of yourself.
2. Reduce body fat. Getting rid of any excess body fat stored in your body.
3. Improve muscle tone and definition. You will appear more physically lean, toned and well-defined.
4. Increase your level of physical attractiveness to others.
5. Many other related benefits.

Health:

1. Reduce blood pressure, reducing your chances of developing hypertension.
2. Increase muscular strength and coordination. Improve ability to function in daily tasks and demands.
3. Strengthen bones. Physical activity, particularly walking, running and resistance exercises can aid the bone strengthening process that naturally occurs within our bodies throughout our life.
4. Improve immune system function. Greatly reduces susceptibility to, and severity of, colds, illnesses and other diseases.
5. Reduce risk of developing various types of cancers as you age. If you have any present cancers, you could slow down the potential development and aid in their management.
6. Many other related benefits.

Wellbeing:

1. Increase your daily energy levels and physical presence.
2. Increase the clarity of your thinking and mental focus.
3. Produce within yourself a greater sense of calm, peace and contentment.
4. Increase your overall levels of self-esteem and confidence.
5. Contribute to the building and maintaining of a positive mental attitude.
6. Aid any sleep problems and improve your overall quality of sleep.
7. Give you a powerful feeling of control over your life which could develop your character, personal pride and happiness.
8. Many other related benefits.

What could happen if you don't change anything?

Physique:

1. Increase potential for weight gain.
2. Increase potential for increase in body fat.
3. An underdeveloped, weak looking physical appearance.
4. Not looking your best or living life in your best physical shape.

Health:

1. Increase your potential for developing cardiovascular diseases.
2. Increase the possibility of experiencing a stroke, now or later in your life.
3. Increase your chances of developing type 2 diabetes.
4. Increase your chances of developing some types of cancer.
5. Loss of fertility or reduced sexual performance.
7. Increase your chances of developing osteoarthritis and other various joint pains.
8. Many more forms of sickness and diseases.

Wellbeing:

1. Loss of self-esteem.
2. Increase your levels of anxiety and timidity.
3. Feel fatigued more regularly.
4. Could lead to depression or loss of enthusiasm for life.
5. Boredom. Lack of challenge and productive activity in your life.
6. Reduced brain function and mental focus.
7. Many more other related consequences.

"Shallow men believe in luck, strong men believe in cause and effect."
– Ralph Waldo Emerson

Just Decide

Ultimately the more you like and respect yourself as a person, the more you will understand the vital importance that your health plays in your life. Our health really is the foundation upon which we build our lives. The starting point for losing weight and achieving a very high level of health and wellbeing is simply to decide to do it. Everything begins with a single firm and definite decision.

"It's not where we stand but in what direction we are moving."
– Johann Wolfgang von Goethe

Action Step Implementation:

Make the Decision.
You're either in or you're out. You cannot take a half-hearted approach to improving your life. You must firmly resolve that you're not going to look back, give up or change course.

Decide, commit and succeed.

If you're serious, then read on. If not, then it's probably best for you to just focus on the areas of your life that you are truly committed to.

"To every action there is always opposed an equal reaction."
– Isaac Newton

YES / NO
(Circle your choice)

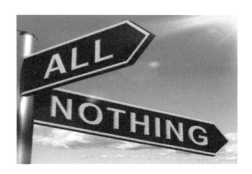

-2-

How Weight and Fat Loss works

Losing Weight and Body Fat is a Skill

Losing weight and body fat is actually quite a simple process, yet for some it feels anything but. There are a few fundamental points that you have to understand to be successful.

In this chapter I will make you aware of the main determining factor that's responsible for whether or not you will lose, gain or maintain your body's weight. Your ability to drop the pounds is completely in your own hands and once you begin to learn and truly understand, you will burn away excess body fat at a rapid rate. This is a skill that can be learned by anyone and applied at any time in your life.

Once you gain experience through your own practice, you'll acquire the skill of estimating your current state of energy balance at any given time, which you will then be able to measure and determine whether or not you're on track with losing weight.

Why We Accumulate Excess Body Fat

It's intuitive; eat more calories than you burn, you gain weight. This is called *positive energy balance*. Eat fewer calories than you burn, you lose weight. This is called *negative energy balance*. Excess calories have got to go somewhere so they get stored as extra body weight in the form of fat. However there are other factors and triggers that contribute to this process that I'd like you to understand.

We all have a set number of predetermined fat storing cells within our bodies. It's the *size* of these cells that varies from person to person not the actual number. Picture these cells as lots of little balloons inside your body, under your skin and around your vital organs. When you are in a positive energy balance, the excess calories are transported into these fat cells causing them to grow, much like inflating a balloon. If you are in a state of negative energy balance i.e. a caloric deficit, this results in the fat being released (to be broken down for energy) much like air let out of a balloon, and so the fat reduces.

For long-term weight loss then it's clear you need to **consistently achieve a negative energy balance.** Daily physical activity and exercise act as a helper to deflate these balloons and release more air each day, hence accelerating the weight loss process. The size of these balloons or cells clearly determines our physical appearance. There is no doubt that how we look impacts on our confidence, i.e. how we feel about ourselves.

The other thing I need you to be aware of is the fat storage promoting hormone, *insulin*. Foods rich in carbohydrates increase blood sugar and since this needs to be maintained within a narrow range, it triggers the release of insulin – the hormone whose primary function is regulating energy and blood sugar. Insulin is released from the pancreas into the bloodstream.

The function of insulin is to lower blood sugar levels and it does this by facilitating the uptake of excess sugar into cells through molecular changes on the surface of the cells. So in effect they 'grab hold' of whatever excess energy they can. Excess sugar is turned into fat and stored (the inflating balloon). The **type** of food you eat therefore impacts directly on how much is stored as fat.

"A moment on the lips, forever on the hips."
– Unknown

The Law of Energy Balance/ Thermodynamics

The only factor that will determine whether you lose weight, put on weight or stay the same *is the state of energy balance* within your body. Everything is energy.

The Law of Thermodynamics, stated simply, says that at the end of every day we will maintain our current body weight, gain weight or lose weight in accordance with the balance of energy in our body. Body fat, however, works slightly differently since other factors are involved. These will be discussed later. However for losing weight and reducing body fat you must recognise, learn and consciously put yourself into a negative state of energy balance every day.

I have created a specific system, or way of living, which will ensure you achieve this goal. This system will be explained fully in Chapter 11. But first it's essential you understand the biology of weight loss and gain.

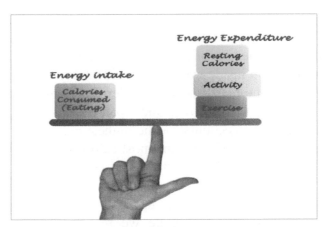

Figure 1: Energy Balance

Energy In

To make sure this is easy to understand I will break it down into its simplest form. Every time we eat or drink, we take calories into our body. A calorie is a *unit measurement of energy.*

Since not all foods are created equal, some foods, that we'll call the 'bad foods', don't give us many of the essential nutrients our body needs in relation to the higher amounts of energy, or calories they contain per gram, *we must eat less of these.* In contrast, the 'good foods' provide essential nutrients, but since they contain less energy or calories per gram, *we can eat more of them*. You will develop a good understanding about the types of food and the calorie/energy values in the next chapter. This will enable you to make smart choices that will aid your weight and fat loss efforts.

How we use this energy depends on various factors. All processes within the body need energy but different processes require different amounts and we can train our bodies to use energy more efficiently as you will see.

> *"One should eat to live, not live to eat."*
> **– Moliere**

Energy Out

Our RMR or Resting Metabolic Rate, otherwise known as our metabolism, is *the amount of energy our bodies need simply to stay alive*. Every function inside every cell, inside every tissue, that make up every organ in the body, use energy derived from food; from the beating of our hearts to the growth and repair of cells.

Our metabolism accounts for the highest portion of the energy we consume every day. This means most calories are used simply to maintain life. Around 65% – 75% of the energy burned from our foods is used in this way.

However, it is possible to increase the rate at which we naturally burn those calories while we rest, and that is through exercise; particularly some of the resistance or weight training exercises that I will show you later.

Exercise will raise your RMR by increasing the amount of lean muscle tissue being built and maintained throughout your body and this tissue requires more energy to maintain than normal tissue. So even when you have stopped working out for the day, your increased RMR means you still burn more calories.

Our Daily Movement Level

From walking, to talking, to clicking our fingers we need energy. Every physical movement or action we take, no matter how small, requires a small amount of energy and this is derived from food. This is only a *very small part* of our daily energy output in relation to how much our metabolism demands from us, but it's still important.

Our Daily Physical Activity Level

This is *the amount of exercise and physical activity we perform each day*. Exercise requires a lot more energy than the simple daily movements outlined above; therefore it's one of the most important *contributors* to shifting energy balance to achieve the desired negative state needed for weight loss and reduction of body fat.

TEF

The Thermic Effect of Food (TEF) is *the amount of energy used by the body for processing the food we eat* (digestion, assimilation etc.) and is another factor that uses up a *relatively small amount* of our daily total energy. Essentially it's the energy needed to break down, digest and transport the foods we eat around our bodies to be used.

Different types of foods require more energy to digest than others, so you can affect your energy balance by *choosing* the foods you eat. High quality lean protein for example is something I will suggest you include in every meal and I will explain why in the next chapter.

But do note that the energy expenditure or TEF is also *very small*. So don't rely on this method too much while trying to lose weight and body fat. However if you understand the differences, you can learn to maximise the thermic effect of different foods by making the right choices. Figure 2 is a chart that outlines the different ways in which we use the food or calories we put into our bodies on a daily basis. It provides a rough estimate of how each one impacts on our balance of energy at the end of each day. Note that this is provided more as a *general idea*; the exact percentages are different for everybody.

Energy Out Factors

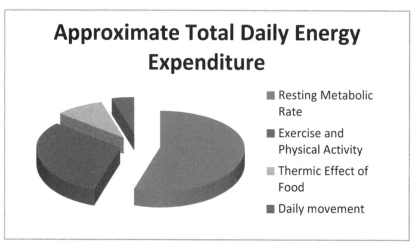

Figure 2: Energy Expenditure

What this information does is show you what we need energy for and so how this must be factored into our weight loss programme. **The primary focus has to be what we eat.** We need to eat highly nutritious foods which give us all the fuel and nutrients we need, yet keeping the total calorie or energy intakes in check.

We will incorporate physical activity and exercise to increase the rate at which we lose weight and body fat and in doing so also nicely sculpt our bodies. A more attractive shape builds confidence.

Table 1 summarises the energy balance we have talked about; but you have to make sure you keep this in mind to succeed on your programme. Your goal is to become aware, understand and then develop the habit of putting yourself into an overall negative state by the end of each day in order to lose weight. And once you reach your desired goal then balance this so that you neither lose nor gain weight. What you don't want is a positive energy balance as this means weight gain.

The Common Denominator in all successful weight loss is achieving a negative energy balance.

Energy IN > Energy OUT	= Weight Gain
Energy IN ⬌ Energy OUT	= Weight Maintenance
Energy IN < Energy OUT	**= Weight Loss**

Table 1: The Energy Balance of Weight Loss, Gain or Maintenance

The Determining Factor

The relationship between the amount of calories we eat in our diet and the amount of energy we use in the body, defines our body weight and our state of physical health.

What goes into the mouth increases the balance of energy. The amount and type of exercise incorporated into our lifestyle decreases the balance of energy. It should always be your goal to **establish a slight negative energy balance every day** to keep losing weight and burning off excess body fat simultaneously.

Avoid starving yourself or only eating tiny amounts as this can be counterproductive. However, by slightly reducing your intakes over time and keeping physically active you will be making progress daily towards the leanest and thinnest version of you.

"Success is the sum of small efforts, repeated day in and day out."
– Robert J Collier

The Difference between Body Weight and Body Fat

We tend to think that losing weight just means losing fat by eating less and exercising more, but actually body weight and how we lose it is not just about body fat levels. Body weight is the total weight of muscle, fascia, bones etc. and exercise does not only lose fat, it can build or even reduce muscle, depending on the nature of the exercise.

This means weight loss is dynamic and body fat loss is dependent on a few factors. *One of these is the kind of foods we eat,* hence the expression: *you are what you eat*. This is explained in more detail in the next chapter.

Our physique is an outward reflection of the quality and quantity of food we eat every day. And for many of us it's the changes we see to our physique that create the drive to keep going when we start to lose weight. This change is also affected by *how much* we exercise and the *type* of exercise we do.

By including resistance or weight training, for example, you will lose fatty tissue and replace it with lean, firm muscle which is denser than fat and therefore changes our body shape. So while eating a healthy, nutritious, clean diet will be your main tool to good health and weight loss, you will achieve the greatest results and make the fastest changes to your physique when you invest a small amount of time in a few key exercises every day.

Six-pack Abs or Six-pack Slabs?

Many believe that daily repetitions of sit-ups and crunches will help us to develop a nice set of abdominal muscles: *cheese grater abs*. This however is *just not true*. Even with all these crunches, no matter how hard you work, your abs are unlikely to be visible unless you have very little body fat.

Until you reduce this body fat to around *ten percent for men* and *fifteen percent for women* you will not see them. The only way to lose the fat and see the muscle is to create that slightly *negative energy balance* each day and of course the only way to do that is by controlling what you eat and when you eat it.

> *"Nothing tastes as good as feeling thin feels."*
> **– Unknown**

Develop your Energy-Balance Awareness

With time and practice you can learn to assess the state of energy balance your body is in. Begin by working out your daily starting point. Make sure what you eat each day is scheduled so it becomes habitual. By eating at the same times each day, around the same amount of food of a similar kind, you can start to *estimate* how much you are taking in each day.

By appreciating how much energy is contained in the various food types you consume, then the more discerning you can be about choice, and how those choices impact on your energy balance. Getting into this slightly negative energy balance will also require some understanding of the processes inside your body. Initially you will need to deal with feeling uncomfortable at certain points of your day.

This discomfort may come in the form of slight hunger; having to use willpower to refrain from bad habits and wrong food choices. Yet with time this feeling will become far less noticeable, because you will have developed a new way of eating and using energy.

So, from this starting point, your goal each day must be to reduce the portions, increase the amount of great quality, highly nutritious foods and eliminate as much of the high calorie unhealthy food as you can. Developing your energy-balance awareness is a *skill* that develops with experience. In the next chapter you will learn all the right foods to eat and to avoid, and how and when to eat for best results.

> *"None of us can change our yesterdays but all of us can change our tomorrows."*
> **– Colin Powell**

-3-

Nutrition

Nutrition is the Key

While genetics may influence our body shape, the tendency to gain weight and where and how we distribute body fat, it is **not an excuse** for overeating and weight gain, it just might mean some people have to work harder than others to achieve the physique and the healthy life they desire.

What we eat and when we eat is important and the saying "Eat less, exercise more", while good advice, is simply not enough on its own. There are a variety of factors and principles that are vital to adhere to when it comes to eating to lose weight. Some of these factors are very simple such as *how, when, why, what* to eat.

So it's a case of changing from unproductive ways of doing this by losing the bad habits we've picked up over the years. This is achieved through re-education; finding out which foods to eat and when. The time of the day and types of foods we eat is also very important and yet is so often disregarded.

All Food is Energy, Yet Produces Different Results

Nutrients are vital for all complex cellular level processes within the body. To simplify and focus this discussion I will explain the main function of each key nutrient in relation to weight loss, burning fat and building a lean physique: the leaner, fitter, healthier you.

Protein

Protein is the nutrient responsible for the growth, repair and maintenance of body tissues, particularly our lean muscle tissue. When we eat high quality foods containing protein, we consume approximately 4kcals of energy per gram.

But it's the high thermic effect of protein that is most significant for weight loss, with approximately 20–35% of calories being burned through digesting and transporting the nutrients in your body. So by ensuring all meals contain a high amount of lean protein you will facilitate weight loss.

Since proteins are used for the building and repair of lean muscle tissue, a high amount of lean protein every day, will also ensure you build and maintain lean muscle tissue in favour of fatty tissue.

Sources of Lean Protein to include in your diet:

1. **Lean Poultry:** chicken, turkey and other game meats (always cut off fat/skin)
2. **Fresh Fish:** salmon, haddock, tuna, cod and other types of fresh fish (wild caught)
3. **Lean Meats:** poultry, lamb, pork and other types of lean meats (always cut off the fat)
4. **Omega-3 Eggs** (Specifically the egg whites)
5. **Protein containing low fat dairy products:** Low fat natural plain yoghurt, low-fat cottage cheese (eat dairy sources of protein in *small amounts* only as they are higher in calories)
6. **Protein Supplements:** protein powders such as whey or casein protein powder. High quality protein bars.

If by any chance you happen to be a vegetarian, this has no limiting affect whatsoever on your ability to build and hold onto a well-defined, lean looking physique. There are many foods that are eaten by vegetarians that also include high quality lean proteins; here are some examples:

Vegetarian Sources of Lean Protein to include in your diet:

- Tofu
- Soy products
- Tempeh
- Omega-3 Eggs. (Specifically egg whites)
- Chickpeas
- Low-fat dairy products such as plain natural yoghurt and low-fat cottage cheese (eat in *smaller amounts* due to being higher in calories)
- Protein supplements: vegetarian protein powders such as egg, pea, hemp, potato.
- Vegetables containing protein such as sweet potatoes & spinach
- Legumes

If you're a vegetarian, it would be a good investment of your time to research online or buy a good quality book on sources of proteins that you could include in your diet as well as how to mix your meals up into tasty, balanced meals.

Carbohydrates

Carbohydrates are *our main fuel source*; the simplest breakdown product being glucose and this is used to drive every cellular reaction in the body. Of course we need it to fuel all our physical activity including exercise. It's important for us consume high quality carbohydrates and to remember that consuming an excess of carbohydrate will result in it being taken up and converted into fat.

It's for that reason we need to eat the *right types* of carbohydrate at the *right times* of the day for optimal digestion (see later). The heavier, starchy carbohydrates that tend to cause fatigue and promote fat storage must be avoided or eaten only on occasion, whereas fibrous carbohydrates, such as vegetables have a much lower insulin spike and fat storage potential, that's why these are the ones we want to consume more often.

Thinking of your carbohydrates in terms of *energy* means you can make a better judgement of when is a good time to eat. Consider that at certain times of the day you need more *energy;* the prime example being first thing in the morning when sugar levels will be at their lowest or before a high intensity training session.

Conversely at night time, when you come home from all your day's activities, you should *limit* carbohydrates as they are more likely to put you into a positive energy balance and be stored as fat, so this is the time when you should favour protein over carbohydrate.

Interestingly, carbohydrates, like proteins, provide us with 4kcals of energy per gram, but the difference is they have a much lower thermic effect with only about 5–15% of the total calories being used in their processing hence it's easy to have an excess. For carbohydrates I will teach you the *right kinds* to consume as well as *when to eat them* to put to good use and avoid being stored as extra body fat.

Sources of quality carbohydrates for you to include in your meals daily:

1. **Fresh fruits** such as: mixed berries (strawberries, blueberries, raspberries, etc.), oranges, grapefruits, tangerines, mandarins, pineapples, papayas, mangoes, kiwi fruit, cherries, lemons, limes, grapes, apples, pears, peaches, plums, melons (galia melon, cantaloupe, honeydew, watermelon), bananas **(eat in smaller amounts)**
2. **Fresh vegetables** such as spinach, lettuce varieties (baby gem, iceberg, romaine, mixed leaves), broccoli, cauliflower, cabbage, green beans, peas, carrots, parsnips, celery, beetroot, tomatoes, radishes, pumpkin, butternut squash, mixed peppers, mushrooms, brussel sprouts, garlic, onions, spring onions, cucumbers, fresh herbs (coriander, basil, parsley, dill, chives, etc.) **(eat in larger amounts)**
3. **Higher density unrefined carbohydrates** like 100 percent whole grains, such as: oats, oatmeal, brown whole-grain rice, whole-grain barley, quinoa **(eat in smaller amounts)**

4. **Sweet potatoes (in smaller amounts)**

Carbohydrates and their Effect on Fat storage

Carbohydrates, shortly after consumed, release glucose into our blood which triggers the release of the hormone, insulin. Insulin is the hormone responsible for controlling blood sugar levels and fat storage within the cells of our body.

The starchier and less natural the carbohydrates we eat (heavy pastas, bread, wheat products, processed foods) with what we call a (**high GI index**); the more insulin is released into our bloodstream. It's this insulin spike, as you know, that increases the potential for fat storage. In general, the more body fat a person has overall, especially around their waist area, the poorer their body's response to insulin over time from these foods and the higher the risk of developing type 2 diabetes. The lighter the carbohydrates we eat a (**low GI index**) such as those found in vegetables and fruits, the smaller the spike and the less likely we are to store it as fat.

So put simply, to aid weight loss *avoid the high GI heavier carbohydrates and focus on the lower GI, fibrous carbohydrates* in fruit and vegetables. Of course there will be times when you will eat the heavier carbohydrates, but my advice is to eat them in the morning as fuel for the day and if consumed early it means they are more likely to be used as energy and not stored as fat.

A good example would be to have a bowl of oatmeal porridge for your breakfast, with its accompanying piece of fruit and yoghurt. As a light lunch you could consider whole-grain pasta, protein, vegetables and a light pasta sauce but try to *avoid these heavy carbohydrates after 2pm*, especially during the evening as they are more likely to be stored as fat.

Choose Whole-grain over Whole-wheat

Whole-grain cereals, pastas, rice, tortillas etc. are much better for you to consume than whole-wheat or white flour products. This is because whole-grain products are not refined like whole-wheat and white flour carbohydrates and therefore still contain all their natural nutrients and are free of toxins and chemicals accumulated in whole-wheat and white flour refining.

One hundred percent whole-grain products are also much lower in fat content but their bulk leaves us feeling fuller. Whole-grains also produce a slightly lower spike in blood glucose levels, which can reduce fat storage.

Balance Your Meals

A good rule of thumb when eating carbohydrates is to *never eat them in a meal alone.* When we consume a high amount of high GI starchy carbohydrates by themselves we have nothing to provide an alkaline load that helps to balance out the glucose and therefore our blood glucose levels can rise to extremely high levels, causing our insulin levels to spike dramatically and we store excess body fat as a result.

By *balancing* your carbohydrate meals with protein, fruit or vegetables, you provide an alkaline load to the blood, which reduces the blood glucose level and the affects that the hormone insulin may cause in fat storage.

Fats

Fat is essential and needed for a wide variety of functions including maintenance of our organs as well as things like hormone production. However we only need *small amounts* from the food we eat daily. There are also *different types* of fats which I will explain to you in detail below. Here is what you need to know about each one:

Omega-3 Polyunsaturated Fats

Omega-3 polyunsaturated fatty acids are fats which cannot be produced by our body and therefore are *essential* and required from food sources or an omega-3 supplement such as fish or flax oil.

These fats improve the health and functioning of our joints, skin, eyes, lungs, heart, hormones, cells and brain development. They also serve to reduce our cholesterol levels, blood pressure, inflammation, while simultaneously encouraging fat burning within the cells of our body.

When combined with a good eating routine and exercise, they will help to *promote* weight and fat loss. Foods we gain these omega-3 fats from are: wild-caught fresh oily fish such as salmon, sardines, tuna, herring, anchovies, halibut, scallops, mussels. Omega-3 is also present in walnuts, ground flaxseed, avocado and some other food sources.

If you dislike eating any of the foods mentioned above, your best choice would be to visit your local health store and invest in a high quality credible omega-3 fish oil supplement. You can find out more about these in the supplement chapter later in this book. If you're a vegetarian or don't like to eat fresh oily fish, consider including some ground flaxseed into your meals or supplement with a flaxseed oil. This is the plant version you could use to increase your essential omega-3s and all their excellent health promoting benefits.

The thermic effect of consuming fats is very low compared to proteins, with only 2% of the total calories being burned in their digestion and assimilation. It's best not to think of eating fats for their thermic effects and instead think of them *for achieving optimal health and promoting fat burning and weight loss.*

Omega-6 Monounsaturated Fats

Omega-6 monounsaturated fats are also known as 'good fats' because they provide a wide range of health benefits, aiding and improving many of the functions required by our body when consumed in **small amounts.** The main sources of omega-6 fats include: nuts, seeds, vegetable oils.

However, too many monounsaturated fats can be counterproductive so again it is all about achieving a balance. Most of us consume too many monounsaturated fats and neglect or simply do not get enough omega-3 polyunsaturated fats to balance these omega-6 fats out.

Saturated Fats

You should ensure the saturated fats you eat come from lean cuts of meat and low-fat dairy products. We only need a *very small amount* of these fats daily to promote brain, organ and hormone function.

Trans Fats

Avoid and strive to completely eliminate trans fats from your diet. This type of fat will cause you to gain excess body fat, ruin your weight loss efforts and lead to all associated health problems and diseases.

Fats Summarised and Getting the Balance Right

We want to aim for a nice *balance* of saturated fats, omega-3 fats and omega-6 fats and avoid or completely eliminate the trans fats contained in processed foods. Good fats, also known as the essential fatty acids (EFAs) cannot be produced by our bodies and therefore we must ingest them from a dietary source or supplement.

However, too many of these fatty acids can also have adverse effects. That's why it's important to strike the **right balance,** particularly between omega-3 and omega-6 fatty acids. Today the majority of us have an imbalance of these two fats, consuming far too much omega-6 in comparison to omega-3 with ratios as high as 20:1 in favour of omega-6.

This can be harmful to the physique and the overall health. It can promote excess oestrogen and bring about metabolic disorders. These conditions can result in excess fat storage in areas like the chest, thighs and hips in men. This can also increase vulnerability to some cancers, as well as causing inflammation and swelling around our joints from overconsumption of omega-6 fats without the anti-inflammatory aid from the omega-3 fats.

We want to make it our goal to tip this ratio more towards *4:1 – 1:1*, (omega-6: omega-3). Never get too caught up in the exact ratios, instead just be intent and focused on consuming more omega-3 in your diet or invest in a fish or flax oil supplement. This will tip the balance of omega 3:6 in your favour and avoid all the negative effects outlined.

The omega-6 fats will come to you naturally from your diet, so there is no need to supplement or intentionally eat foods containing them.

What To Eat (Building your Daily Meals)

What you eat is one of the biggest influences you will have on how you look and the quality of your health throughout your life. **Your diet is the key.** When I speak of the term diet, I'm not referring to eating a set of specific foods for a certain period of time in order to lose weight and look good; I mean the food that you eat, day to day. As you know a little more about the different nutrients derived from your foods, you now need to understand that you need to eat more of some of them and less of the others – if your goal is to keep losing weight.

Protein always comes first. In every meal of the day: breakfast, lunch and your evening meal, including any snacks, **make protein the basis.** Picture your bowl or plate, what kind of lean protein are you going to have in this meal?

Once you have a good amount of lean, quality protein, you can then choose some carbohydrates to accompany it, and in some meals, if possible, a small amount of good healthy omega-3 fat. Protein is the *first* and *most essential part* of each of your daily meals. Remembering **that we are what we eat,** by eating lean protein in each meal, we will always be maintaining lean muscle tissue keeping our body in a constant state of fat burning and lean tissue recycling.

High quality proteins also keep us fuller for longer, allowing us to function and perform for longer between each of our daily meals. Once we have a good amount of quality protein in our meal, then we can add our carbohydrates. *Fibrous lighter carbs* such as vegetables are your ultimate choice for weight and fat loss.

They are very low in calories, yet high in nutrients. This allows us to eat more of them in comparison to other heavier, starchy carbohydrates such as bread or pasta. In some meals you can substitute the vegetables for fruits to accompany your proteins. While fruits have all the great nutrients you find in vegetables, they do contain more calories.

That's why you want to *generally eat more vegetables than fruits*, although fruits do make good snacks. Try to eat around a *4:1 or 5:1* ratio of vegetables compared to fruits. Too many fruits can reduce your total fat burning potential due to the higher amounts of sugar you will have in your body.

Also try to avoid eating fruits later at night; make a point to consume them earlier in the day so that the natural sugars get used as energy in your daily activities. By including high amounts of vegetables and fruits in our diet every day, we provide ourselves with all the health promoting antioxidants that will go to work in our bodies to fight off and prevent infections, cancers and other diseases. The more brightly coloured the fruit and vegetables, the more antioxidants they contain.

When it comes to fruits, always eat the *whole, fresh fruit versions* over dried fruit. Dried fruits have much higher sugar content and less nutritional value per gram therefore are not good at promoting weight and fat loss. As for healthy fats, if you're not getting them from a supplement each day, add in very small amounts of omega-3 fatty acids.

You can do this by including some fresh fish with your lunch or evening meal or mixing some ground flaxseed into your oatmeal porridge or mixed fruit salad. In the chapter on cooking and recipes, I will provide more than enough examples and ideas of how to mix up these meals efficiently to maximize the balance of nutrients that promote you building an excellent physique.

For now the main thing I want you to take away is that in building each of your meals, try to mix your foods up into tasty, balanced nutritious meals *using fresh, whole, single ingredient foods.*

Always remember the rule of protein first, vegetables second, then some fruit, some healthy omega-3 fats, and some other recommended high quality carbohydrates.

Understand the Nutrient and Energy Density of your Foods

Some foods provide us many more nutrients than others. Foods I will teach you to avoid will be ones with few nutrients but which overload with excess calories making it very difficult, even impossible, to achieve the desired negative energy balance required for weight and fat loss. That's why I want to teach you how to know the *quality* of the foods you're eating in each meal. There are two factors you must become aware of.

Nutrient Density: Nutrient Density is *the nutrient component of food*; nutrients being essential for fuel, growth and repair of muscle tissues and other essential functions. Nutrients include vitamins, minerals, phytonutrients, fibre, fats, carbohydrates and lean proteins. Some foods contain very high levels of nutrients per gram. An example would be a large salad, also low in calories.

Energy Density: Energy Density is *the energy component of food*. Some foods do not provide us with many beneficial nutrients but instead overload with excess calories. An example being chocolate biscuits. They may not look like much, but they would load us with calories that would serve us no good purpose.

Practice Carbohydrate Swapping

Carbohydrate swapping is one of the easiest and most effective methods you could use in dropping your body fat levels and losing lots of weight in a short period of time. Not only that, but it may even be more beneficial for your overall health, energy and vitality.

Basically you simply replace all the higher density, starchy carbohydrates you normally eat throughout your day such as breads, pastas, rice, bagels and cereals with *fibrous carbohydrates* such as fresh vegetables and fruits instead.

Fruit and vegetables release a much lower level of blood glucose into our bloodstream, therefore reducing the spikes in our blood glucose and the hormone insulin's effects on storing fat. Fruit and vegetables also provide essential nutrients.

Replace grains with greens and you will greatly accelerate your weight and fat loss, while increasing your intake of fibre and all the other important vitamins and minerals.

Love Your Foods

If the foods you're eating do not taste good to you and you don't enjoy them, modify them. Try out new recipes. Modify and season foods to make them more enjoyable. Learn to create both balanced and nutritious meals that taste great at the same time. This is an *art* you develop through practice.

Summary of What to Eat:

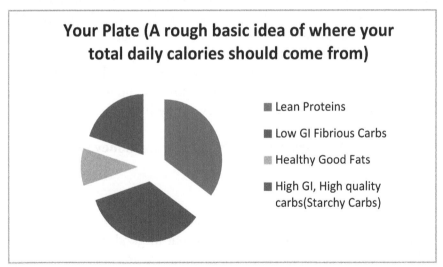

Figure 3: Calorie Breakdown

Figure 3 is only intended as a *guide*; you may have more proteins or vegetables, or no high GI carbs, yet overall achieve a similar balance.

> *"A healthy outside starts from the inside."*
> **– Robert Urich**

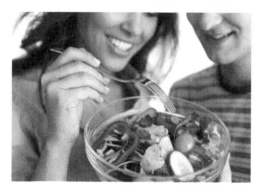

How To Eat

Many of us have forgotten *how to* eat food in the most natural, productive way so that it maximises the experience and enhances the absorption and assimilation of its component nutrients. Today it's rare that we *take the time* to sit down to enjoy our foods and the whole 'eating experience'. We're busy; we eat on the go, often for convenience and therefore don't pay close attention to what we're eating and how that impacts on our everyday lives.

Eating without awareness is like throwing money in the bin.

The Eating Process

You need to train yourself to eat *only when you're hungry* so that food is always absorbed fully and put to good use. Sadly many of us have very poor habits of eating when we are not really hungry. If the body is not sending the signal that we require food then in every likelihood that food will be excess and therefore stored as body fat.

This would be a waste of money, food, time and even harmful to the organs of our body in the long term. Also train yourself to eat approximately every *four hours* as this is an ideal amount of time between meals. Maximise the eating experience: have a seat, take your time and enjoy what you're eating.

Be fully present in the moment and focused on what you're eating. Eating should never be a peripheral activity while watching TV, talking on the phone or reading a newspaper. Slow down, never rush, avoid all distractions and fully enjoy the whole eating experience.

"Do not dwell in the past; do not dream of the future, concentrate the mind on the present moment."

– Buddha

When To Eat

Tune in to your own Natural Biology
Today, most of us have long forgotten what it truly feels like to experience hunger. Most of us never get any sensations of true physical hunger. We have rushed ahead and eaten our next meal before our bodies have even had the time to fully digest and make use of the previous one.

We need to consciously work to become more in tune with the natural intelligence of our own bodies. We need to recognise when our body is calling out for raw materials in the form of quality nutrients so that it can fuel our body with energy, or repair used up muscle and cell tissues.

Examples of how you can recognise genuine physical hunger include stomach grumbling, feeling a sense of lower energy or fatigue; your taste buds would welcome and enjoy almost any food, not a specific craving for one type in general. It's important that you always eat when you feel physically hungry, but *never starving*.

Being in a state of starvation can be very counterproductive, slowing down our metabolism and decreasing our body's ability to burn fat. It's always good to know and plan your eating ahead of your day so that you don't fall into the undesirable state of starvation at any point. *Listening* to your body is a *skill* that once you get in sync with, will become a natural part of your way of eating.

> *"Intelligence is present everywhere in our bodies... our own inner intelligence is far superior to any we can try to substitute from the outside."*
> **– Deepak Chopra**

A Good Daily Meal Plan Example

A basic, yet very effective, plan for your meals and eating looks like this: a moderate sized, high quality breakfast to kick-start your metabolism and fuel your body, your brain and harness the energy required for the long day and its challenges ahead. It will ensure that you function at your best; it will *light your fire* first thing in the morning and keep it going throughout the day.

Around four hours later, when lunchtime comes around, have a highly nutritious lunch consisting of lean high quality protein and vegetables and even a small amount of starchy carbs such as a whole-grain wrap, pitta, couscous or rice. *Then another four hours later* for your evening meal more high quality protein, plenty of vegetables and a light low fat sauce.

Then if you find yourself hungry again later that night, consider a high quality protein snack to keep those muscles fed and body fat burning away. If at any point between when you awake and go to sleep, you experience a high degree of physical hunger, snack on something like a high quality source of protein and a piece of whole fresh fruit.

The rule is it must include a high quality, lean source of protein every time.

Eating Will Never Solve Emotional Problems

Never eat for emotional reasons. You need to become more aware of all the potential emotional triggers that cause you to turn to food, and then stop yourself acting before you reach for something to eat. Some of these emotional triggers include:

- Stress
- Anger
- Boredom
- Sadness
- To fill a void or something currently missing from your life
- To feel safe and comfortable
- To recapture a high emotional feeling or memory
- As a social activity
- Many others, you find yours

Emotional hunger can never be satisfied with eating food. It will only leave you feeling more negative about yourself and even guilty afterwards. If you happen to fall victim to any kinds of eating for emotional reasons, the first step is *awareness.* Simply become aware of yourself before you turn to eating as a solution.

Once you're aware of the emotional eating pattern, you need to look deeper to *discover the real reason* behind your impulse to choose food. You then need to focus on taking positive action towards a more realistic solution. So start with working towards this awareness; ask yourself when and why you turn to food.

Then you will have more control and power over choosing not to eat or even better, solving the real underlying problem instead. A helpful strategy for people who have a craving for sugary sweets, cakes, drinks or any other products high in sugar would be to catch yourself when you feel compelled to eat one of these and instead of fighting against your body's addiction, give into it by feeding it with a piece of fruit.

Fruit is also high in sugar, the only difference is the quality of sugars are highly nutritious, giving your body the sugars that it's craving, but in the form of *natural sugar*. This will be much more beneficial for weight and fat loss efforts than processed sugars from any form of junk food that will only ruin any hope you may have becoming lean and trim.

The Seven Smaller Meals A Day Concept

Science has taught us that by eating seven smaller meals a day, still containing the same calories as three larger meals, you will burn more fat, and lose a little extra weight, as well as having more energy and feeling stronger. This is because it keeps your metabolism at a constant rate throughout the day, hence burning extra calories at your Resting Metabolic Rate.

While this may be true and I have seen evidence that it works, it is *not necessarily practical*. Unless you're a competing body builder, or a highly active professional athlete, then it would be in your own best interests to forget about the seven smaller meals a day concept.

However if you're interested or have the time and patience for what it demands, feel free to research other books on the subject and try it out in your routine.

Cheat/Treat Meal Concept

Science suggests that having a *cheat meal* every now and again is good for our metabolism and prevents our bodies from thinking that it's being underfed and entering starvation mode, which slows down our metabolism and makes it harder for our bodies to burn fat. This concept is true, yet it is often misunderstood.

The cheat meal should be included in your eating schedule, for psychological, mental and emotional reasons. We want to continue to eat our favourite foods or enjoy eating out and having whatever we choose. However we must make this a *rare event*. One cheat meal a week would be a good rule. Or two smaller cheat snacks.

Make it your goal to reward yourself at the weekend with a meal of your own choice, and a slightly larger portion than usual. But this should be seen as a *reward* given only if you have stayed disciplined to your plan throughout the week of good eating and exercise.

Once you have enjoyed this cheat meal and savoured the moment, get back to your strict focus on achieving your best weight and best body definition, and stay focused until you have earned another cheat meal. Don't have more than one cheat meal each week, or destroy all your hard work by splurging out on junk over the bulk of the weekend.

The main reason I encourage you to treat yourself to one larger, less nutritious meal during the weekend is for the direct benefits on your mental health and motivation. After enjoying a *dirty* meal for a change, you will feel human again. Enjoy the experience while it lasts, feel proud of your efforts and discipline to your good eating and exercise habits. Afterwards you may even begin to feel guilty and look forward to eating a clean, healthy, nutritious meal.

Missed Meals

If at any time you have been so busy that you missed one of your meals or high protein snacks, *don't sweat it*. Just make sure to eat a high quality, nutritious meal as soon as you can, then get back on track again. Be sure that you do not make this a habit, as constantly putting your body into starvation mode can cause metabolic problems, greatly slowing down your metabolism therefore reducing your body's ability to burn fat and get the weight off in the long term.

Quit the Evening Eating

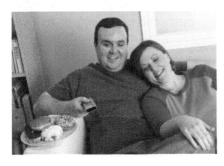 You don't need as much energy to relax in the evening, so you don't need to eat as much as at other times of the day; it's that simple. So cut out all the snacks after your final meal. The only exception

would be if you're experiencing true physical hunger or having problems with getting to sleep due to the natural effects of being in this state of negative energy balance. In this case have a high quality protein snack to feed the muscles that are calling out for food.

How Much to Eat

Every time you eat a meal you need to eat *the right amount*. You don't want to become lethargic and tired as a result of over eating, or continuously think about and look for food by under eating. Again it's about balance. Make it a rule to eat a moderate to large sized meal, made up mostly from low calorie food such as vegetables and a generous serving of protein. You should always end the meal feeling well fed, but not bloated. Strive to be *80% full*.

With time and experience in preparing and cooking your own meals, you'll soon find the perfect balance for you, enough to be happily fed, yet never overdoing it. It may require you to develop a little self-discipline, but after stopping bad unproductive habits of overeating, you will soon find a new normal amount of food to eat.

Low Activity Days

On the days you know ahead of time you are definitely going to be less active or on non-exercise days, make sure that you eat a little less in each meal. Check with your physical activity schedule to decide if you're going to have a lighter eating day.

As We Age

As we age we tend to become less active and more prone to weight gain as our metabolic rate slows. We must therefore *adapt* to this change by *consuming fewer calories and being more active.*

Family and Social Events

Social gatherings will always be a challenge to weight loss programmes so we need to learn to refrain from second helpings and to pass on the dessert. Shift your focus to enjoying these events and spending quality time with family and friends and **don't make food the focus.**

Avoid the Reward Trap

A common misconception is that lots of exercise gives you license to eat what you like and as much as you like. But all this does is stop you achieving your negative energy balance. So don't undo all your hard work!

What Not to Eat

When choosing foods to eat from the supermarket, or buying on the go, always remind yourself: *"Did this food come from a tree or other plant. Is it out of the ground, did it walk, fly or swim?"* If not, then don't put it into your body.

Our healthy, strong, lean ancestors ate from a menu consisting of only hunting and gathering. Now in the 21st century we eat wheat, salt, sugar, chemicals, toxins and high Trans-fats containing products that are silently destroying our health and adding the weight and body fat onto our figures. Here are some things to avoid:

The Three White Poisons

Salt, sugar and **white flour products.**
All three of these act as 'poisons' and are making us fat and robbing us of our health and vitality. Most of us don't avoid them because *we have a short term mind-set.* We may eat a large cake and box of chocolates, feel a little sick, maybe gain a small amount of weight that we feel we can easily take off again sooner or later. However we have to change our thinking to *consider the long term* health problems that result from eating these foods.

The Law of Cause and Effect is always working.

Avoid putting **salt** on food as there is already sufficient natural salt in food to supply your daily sodium needs. Excess can harm your heart, other organs and cause your body to gain weight and store excess body fat. Sugar is addictive and compels us to eat more and more. It is the cause of many health problems.

Sugar is also the main ingredient responsible for shifting our bodies into the fat storage mode and holding onto most of the food we eat, completely shutting down our natural ability to burn fat and lose weight.

White flour is highly refined and has been loaded with chemicals and toxins in the manufacturing process. We have already seen its negative effect on our metabolism and fat storage via *insulin*. If we can *become aware* of what are buying and eating every day, we will soon learn to avoid these poisons and their harmful effects.

What to completely avoid and eliminate from your diet to have any chance of success:

- **Foods containing Trans fats:** baked goods, fried foods, packaged foods, cookies, crackers, biscuits, pies, pastries, desserts, doughnuts, chocolates, etc.
- **The skin or fat** on any of your meats, poultry or fish.
- **Bagged or packaged** chemical containing fruit or vegetables. Prepare them all from fresh yourself.
- **High fat oils.** Such as vegetable oils, corn oil, sunflower oil. These are much higher in calories and may cause harmful inflammation effects within our bodies.
- **Processed foods.** All the foreign substances and chemicals lead to excess body fat gain, sickness, diseases and health problems.
- **High sugar containing foods.**

What to greatly reduce in amounts in order to lose weight and burn more body fat:

- **Butter and margarine.** Very high in unhealthy trans and saturated fats.
- **Nuts, seeds, legumes.** These foods can be beneficial to our health in small amounts, yet the high calorie content is not beneficial in terms of losing weight and body fat.
- **Dried fruits.** These foods can be beneficial to our health in small amounts, yet the high calorie content is not beneficial in terms of losing weight and body fat.
- **Foods high in glucose** that trigger insulin in our bodies. Insulin being the hormone that causes fat storage. High starchy carbohydrates such as pastas, breads, bagels, cereals, rice, etc. mainly products made from flour and wheat.
- **Dairy products.** The high fat content in all dairy products requires that we eat them in small amounts only to put our bodies in the state required for weight and fat loss. **Cheeses, yoghurts, and milks** to be used only in small amounts to complement our meals or tea/coffee and never as a whole meal in itself.

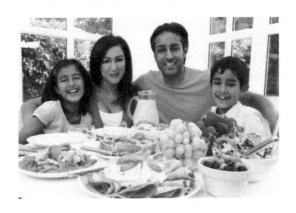

Get Out Of Those Centre Aisles

During your weekly trips to the supermarket, *stay clear of the centre aisles*. These are the aisles that hold all the sugar, flour, salt, Trans fats and highly processed garbage that should not be a part of any healthy human's diet today.

Don't pick up any of these foods that sabotage any chance of your success such as crisps, sweets, pastries, ready-made chemical infested meals, highly refined white flour products, sugary cereals and tinned preserved foods. Make sure that you are only pushing your trolley around the outside aisles of the shop, particularly around the meat, fish, vegetable, fruit and dairy sections for around 80% or more of your entire shopping cart.

Cut Out Liquid Calories

Liquid calories will hold you back from getting into that desired negative energy balance. From fizzy drinks to sweetened coffees or high calorie smoothies and milk shakes, these drinks *go in and out*, providing us with little or no nutritional benefit and they have no satiety value either.

The sugars included in these drinks can actually act as triggers that make us even hungrier than before. There is only one liquid calorie drink that can be beneficial in certain situations: the high quality protein powder and water shake.

This shake should only ever be used as a replacement for a snack, between meals when you are feeling true physical hunger and you intend to feed your muscles and keep the body fat burning. While smoothies and fruit juices may provide some nutritional benefits, they are still very high in sugar content.

Water

Water is the drink *you do* want. Anyone who claims not to like water simply has the wrong attitude towards their health. Water is the fundamental to life. Water should make up the base of everything we drink every day. And *plenty of it.* Throughout the day at regular intervals we should be sipping water as a *habit.*

Water is the most assessable and least costly drink we have on the planet, yet provides us with the most positive benefits. Drinking water keeps us hydrated. It raises our metabolism and flushes out toxins as well as reducing our appetite and hunger levels.

Being fully hydrated also increases mental clarity and focus, and raises our energy levels. As you awake in the morning, you will tend to be in a state of slight dehydration, so start your day with a glass of water, and continue to drink it throughout the day.

At all times, you can know if you're hydrated enough by the colour of your urine. It is clear then you're on the right track. Even up to a two percent dehydration can result in lack of metal focus and physical fatigue.

Green Tea

Another very useful beverage is green tea. Green tea is famous for its *fat burning properties* and it can raise the metabolism for a short time both during and after drinking. Not only is green tea our best friend in losing weight and burning fat, when we consume around *three to five* cups on average each day, there are some remarkable health benefits.

Green tea is full of healthy antioxidants that help us fight diseases, viruses, cancers and keep our immune systems functioning to a high degree. A large mug of green tea before meals can also make you feel fuller – so you eat less.

There is a very small amount of caffeine in green tea that can raise your energy levels, increase your mental clarity and focus and even improve your mood and wellbeing.

Tea/Coffee

For those of you who enjoy a cup of tea or coffee, *keep doing so.* Drinking caffeine in *small* amounts can have helpful effects on stimulating your metabolism and fat burning throughout your day, as well as increasing your focus, productivity and energy levels. However beware; too much has many negative consequences on your health, immune system and wellbeing.

Strive for around two to three smaller cups of tea or coffee over the period of the day if you're a caffeine lover. However do not overdo it or you will be doing yourself more harm than good. If you're currently drinking caffeine in extreme levels, it is advisable to progressively reduce your cups by about one every week and reduce the amounts in each cup until you finally achieve the point where you're consuming a healthy level of around two to three smaller cups a day.

One more rule when it comes to caffeine: *caffeine dehydrates* us, so always remember to also drink water. Don't allow your body to get into a dehydrated state, find the *correct balance* between caffeine and water. Caffeine can be a great tool and pleasure if you use it in the *right amounts* and for the *right reasons*.

All About Alcohol

There is one other fourth source of energy we can give to our bodies that I failed to mention earlier when explaining proteins, carbohydrates and fats. I intentionally missed this one out for a good reason. This fourth source is alcohol. Alcohol provides us with 7kcals of energy for every gram of alcohol we consume.

But these are *empty calories*; they provide little or no nutritional value. When we consume alcohol, we're basically flooding our bodies with all this excess energy that we cannot use for any good purpose. All these additional calories raise our energy balance moving us away from the negative state that we are trying to achieve.

Not only this, but the carbohydrates also included in many alcoholic drinks such as beer or the fizzy drinks we mix with spirits flood our blood with glucose causing the release of the fat storing hormone insulin. The minute we consume alcohol, we cancel out the process of fat burning within our bodies until our body has used up all the energy consumed.

This is because our body has to stop using our stored fats as a source of energy to function and therefore shifts all its attention on breaking down and ridding the body of alcohol before it can then go back to breaking down our fat cells for energy.

Alcohol is known to stimulate the release of cortisol which is a known fat-creating hormone. This hormone works to break down our lean muscle mass and hold on to our stored body fat. Alcohol alone does not directly make us fat; however when taken too frequently over time and in excess, it promotes fat storage in the cells of our bodies and destroys their ability to burn off the body fat.

The negative health effects from alcohol are also numerous, creating a negative impact on our brain function, hydration levels and our overall energy, vitality and wellbeing. Alcohol has no value to us in losing weight and owning a lean, defined physique and only slows down or prevents any progress that we make.

Weight loss and regular alcohol consumption do not mix. My advice on drinking alcohol would be to *save it for special occasions* or one night during the weekend only and to make sure you always consume it in *moderation.* Don't overdo it. The hangover stopping you achieving your physique goals surely isn't worth it.

Have a few drinks, enjoy your nights and special occasions, and yet *know when to stop.* Keep your focus on achieving that body that you have set out to get.

Summary

Your goal and focus should be to develop and maintain a healthy relationship with food for the rest of your life. This means eating clean high quality, natural, whole, nutritious meals, only when you know that you're physically hungry; when your body genuinely needs fuel.

Food should always be used as the tool for energy and growth, repair and maintenance of lean muscle mass that you are currently in the process of building through exercise and physical activity. Make a point to prioritise your life and your time so that you always prepare and cook your own food as much as possible.

One of the single greatest predictors of leanness in a person is the extent in which they eat top quality foods that they have intentionally prepared from the comfort of their own home. Shopping is the key. For anybody who protests that it's hard to eat the right foods, in the right amounts, at the right times, *rethink it* as this overall mind-set will be the secret to your success.

Plan your meals roughly a week in advance, then make sure that you refuse to put anything that is not on your list and supportive of your weight and fat loss efforts into that shopping trolley. What does not make it into your home, cannot be consumed. This is a basic law of human nature.

As humans, we all tend to eat whatever is within our environment. Prevent the possibility of this ever occurring right from the very start by making the habit of putting into that shopping basket of yours only what you would like to represent in your outer physical appearance.

Nutrition, more than any other factor, is the main determinant of your weight loss. Picture yourself as a transparent large tank. What you put into this tank, is exactly what this tank will look like on the outside. You will get out, exactly what you put in. Your physical body today is the sum total of all that you have put into your mouth over the past weeks and months and years.

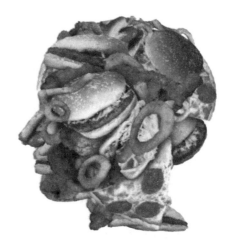

Daily nutrition is the most important component influencing your health and appearance, and accounts for *eighty percent* of your results, whereas exercise is the *tool* influencing the other *twenty percent* of your results, as will be discussed in the following chapter. It is essential that you focus, work hard, understand, learn and live by eating the right foods, at the right times, in the right amounts in the right way.

- Eat a balanced meal around every four hours when you begin to experience symptoms of true physical hunger.
- Make sure that each meal you eat throughout the day contains a source of lean, high quality protein.
- Ensure that you are fully hydrated at all times by consuming water at frequent, regular intervals over the course of your day.
- Ensure that in all meals during the second half of each of your days, after 5pm that you do not eat any starchy carbohydrates, and have only the fibrous carbohydrates instead.
- Prepare and cook your own meals using fresh, whole, natural ingredients. Lots of vegetables, some fruits, lean sources of protein and a small amount of omega-3 good fats.
- Recognise any liquid calories you may be currently consuming in your regular routine and then resolve to eliminate them one by one and cut them out of your diet.
- Eliminate the three white poisons from your house, life and diet. Throw away salt, sugar and all white flour products.

-4-

Exercise

Introduction to Exercise

Learning and living a life of high quality nutritional habits alone is not enough to achieve your physique's full potential and optimise your health. The *tool* that is used to chisel away and mould your body into a strong, lean, well defined, healthy looking figure is an effective routine of regular physical exercise.

We tend to gravitate to one form of exercise over another. We may have past injuries, present health problems or certain disabilities that restrict us and so we must learn to be creative in choosing the right methods and type of exercises. Whatever your current outlook to exercise; whether you love or loath it, you must keep an open mind. Visualise how certain types and ways to exercise can fit into your lifestyle. Focus on finding a way to enjoy the challenge of it.

Exercise is the most basic function and requirement of any human being. We're built to move our bodies but in a 21st century world this is often neglected. Not only does exercise *sculpt you* into the most appealing physique and accelerate weight loss, it also stimulates a feeling of well-being from the release of endorphin hormones.

Exercise, when done in moderation, and sensibly, can assist in the healing of disease, infections, viruses, and even keeps us free from various cancers. It also relieves stress, increases our self-esteem and confidence, and improves our mental capabilities, which means that exercise really is our greatest tool.

Anybody who is currently neglecting their health should seriously consider *investing* as little as a few hours a week engaged in some form of physical exercise. The majority of us today spend around forty to fifty hours sitting at a desk in an office, and then are too mentally and physically exhausted when we get home to exercise.

However, it does not require a huge commitment on your part; you can start with a few short walks every week. As your fitness develops you can build on that with other forms of exercise or longer more frequent walks. The main thing is that you set aside time every week and you'll soon see how much you enjoy it. Don't wait until your health suffers and live to regret not making the changes now.

The Pareto Principle

As a result of exercising in some form or another, every single day of the week, over the past decade, as well as helping a huge variety of clients to achieve their personal health and physique goals during my time as a personal trainer, I have discovered that *there are various specific exercises and techniques that are more effective.*

The Pareto Principle, also known as the 80–20 rule, or the Law of the Vital Few states that, *for many events, roughly 80% of the effects come from 20% of the causes.* An example of this would be in business where 80% of the profits come from 20% of the customers. Or on the job, where 20% of the employees contribute to 80% of the company's results. This 80–20 is also very effective when applied to exercise.

80% of the results in weight loss, fat burning, muscle building and overall physique will result from performing 20% of the exercises. I will show you how you can best apply this to your time spent on exercise to achieve the fastest and greatest results. No more hanging around gyms trying to figure out which exercises are good and which aren't.

No more aimlessly going through the motions trying to perform awkward exercises you see others performing in the weight room. I am going to present you with all the most effective, yet highly functional exercises and methods of exercise from my entire life experience.

To get great rapid and lasting results from working out, it's actually quite *simple,* the problem most of us experience is being overwhelmed – when all we need to do is focus on performing a few select exercises well.

Pre Exercise Warm ups and Movements

Before you begin an exercise session, whether its resistance exercises, weight training, going for a run, getting your lengths done in the pool or practising your skills in a particular sport, it's vital that you *loosen up* the joints and muscles that you will be using during the activity.

This is essential to maximise the benefits of your exercise session and reduce the risks of sprains, strains or even fatal injuries. Therefore it is advisable to undertake a *dynamic warm up* for five to ten minutes (dependent on the nature of the exercise to follow). Your goal is to perform controlled movements at each of the joints in your body that will be used.

For example, if you are about to perform a full body circuit training class, you are likely to be working many muscles therefore it is wise to ensure every joint in your body is prepared. You could start at the top of your body with your neck, performing neck rotations.

After around thirty seconds of neck movements, you would move down to your shoulders, performing circular full arm movements in several different directions and planes of motion. You would then move downwards, loosening up all your other muscles and joints such as your elbows, chest, back, hips, groin, thighs, knees, calves, ankles and so on.

After five to ten minutes of controlled, rhythmic movements you should be ready. *It is also a good idea to perform five to ten minutes of light cardiovascular exercise* such as a light jog, cycle or jumping rope. This increases your heart rate, stimulates your nervous system, lubricates the joints, increases your overall body temperature, warms up your muscles and further prepares you for the demands you're about to place on it.

If the exercise only requires that you exercise your legs and feet, for example running, your pre exercise dynamic warm-up would require only that you spend your time and attention loosening your ankles, knees, hips and groin.

Whatever the exercise activity, it's essential that you always take the time required before you get started, to fully prepare. Don't skip this step. **Your safety always comes first.**

Cardiovascular Exercise

Cardiovascular exercise is an excellent tool for dramatically accelerating weight and fat loss, especially when following great nutritional habits simultaneously. Not only does cardio put your physique onto the fast track, but moderate intensity, aerobic activity is the single most powerful method of exercise to develop a high level of general health and wellbeing.

Regular cardiovascular exercise is the single most important determinant of the state of health. I truly believe that if each one of us incorporates it into our weekly routine, we will quickly see the benefits. A light jog a couple of times each week does wonders for our health. If you can't manage that, a morning walk a few times can be just as beneficial.

Similarly, swimming lengths at your local pool is a wonderful exercise that uses the entire body. Whether walking your dog or running a few miles, the overall message is clear: **cardiovascular exercise promotes optimal physical and mental health.**

There are three different types of exercise that I'm going to discuss in this chapter. 1) Aerobic long steady distance; 2) aerobic interval training and 3) interval training. Each of these three methods of exercise are of different intensities and should be *carefully considered* before implementing them into your routine, depending on your physical capabilities and current fitness level.

Aerobic Long Steady Distance

This is the type of cardiovascular exercise that I recommend most highly of the three. It greatly contributes to our physical and mental health, but has a very low risk of injury or wear and tear in your body and your joints. When we exercise aerobically, we use oxygen as our main source of fuel. Aerobic long steady distance means exercising for a minimum of fifteen minutes, up to one hour.

You don't have to use force to get yourself to work hard; you work at a pace that's comfortable for you. So, you could work at a slow or moderate pace, for a longer duration of time. An example of a slow pace long steady distance workout could be a one hour brisk walk along the beach with the dog.

Another example, this time more of a moderate long steady distance workout, could be having a thirty minute light jog on the treadmill without stopping. Of course you can engage in many other forms of exercise at low or moderate intensity.

For example, using the rowing machine, going for an outdoor cycle, slowly swimming twenty to forty lengths at the swimming pool or using the cross trainer at the gym. The essential element of this type of exercise is the use of *slow to moderate, continuous movement, for longer periods of time* without stopping to take a rest.

The nature of this exercise can be deemed boring for some, particularly if you're at the local gym or health club on a treadmill or another one of the cardiovascular machines. To combat this I highly recommend that you take your mp3 player and listen to music.

Some people prefer to listen to motivational speeches they've downloaded, for others it may be pump up workout music. I listen to relaxing chill out trance style music and the time it takes to complete a thirty minute jog just flies by. Choose what you like to listen to most and create a good playlist to keep you entertained.

If you do your long steady distance exercise on a treadmill or cardiovascular machine at the local gym or health club, the machines you use will have a variety of readings and measurements on them. Don't focus on counting the calories; instead *use the duration* that you maintain your continuous pace of exercise and *the speed you work at.*

You will know if you're improving if you're increasing the speed or duration gradually over time. The more consistently and frequently you perform your long steady distance sessions, the greater the results you will experience in your weight and fat loss efforts and in your overall fitness.

I do long steady cardiovascular exercise around two or three times a week in the form of swimming forty to sixty lengths, or lightly jogging on a treadmill for thirty minutes. As a result, my weight stays at a low trim level, my body fat is kept low and the systems and functions of my body are kept healthy.

Whether you perform three half hour walks a week or go for a couple of bike cycles, it's completely up to you. Generally, running and swimming provide the highest return on your efforts and energy in terms of weight and body fat loss; however any method of cardiovascular training will get you results if you put the time in and remain consistent in your routine.

Don't overdo it, it's not a competition, just do what you can personally get through and *work to improve on your own efforts.*

Aerobic Long Steady Distance Workout Recommendations:

Intensity	Duration
Moderate/Low speed	15-45 m

Table 2

Aerobic Intervals

Aerobic intervals are a slightly more intensive form of cardiovascular exercise that requires a little more effort and energy than the long steady distance method. The main benefit from performing aerobic intervals is the higher return on your health and cardiovascular fitness levels, as well as accelerating your rate of weight and body fat loss.

I have included this method to *widen your options*. If long steady distance aerobic exercise alone becomes tedious you can vary the routine and hence remain motivated. Aerobic intervals are basically the same as long steady distance exercise, where you continue to perform continuous cardiovascular exercise without a break for a set period of time.

However, you would change the speed that you perform the exercise from a slower moderate level, to a moderate level at around two minutes each time. For example you could walk at a moderate pace for a couple of minutes, then speed up and then fast walk for two minutes. Repeat this two minute on and off period around ten times and you have completed a twenty minute aerobic interval walk. This applies also to swimming, where you could swim one length very slowly as a recovery length, then the next at a moderate pace where you expend a little more effort.

You would then repeat this slow and slightly faster length swapping until you have completed around twenty to forty lengths in total. Similarly, and the most common method used by exercisers today, is performing your aerobic intervals on the treadmill. You would set the speed level on the treadmill at a specific determined level, let's say level 5.5 and then jog for two minutes at a slower to moderate pace.

After those two minutes, you would increase the speed level to about 6.5 and then jog for another two minutes at a more moderate pace. Continue this for around ten to fifteen intervals of two minutes at each speed and then you will have completed your aerobic interval session.

Again, the method you use for your aerobic intervals is limited only by your imagination and equipment/facilities available to you. The key is to choose what you most *enjoy* doing, so that you can adhere to this as a part of your weekly routine. Don't let it become a chore.

Aerobic Intervals Workout Recommendations:

Work Intensity	Rest Intensity	Work Duration	Rest Duration	Total Work Sets
Moderate speed	Low/Moderate speed	1-2 (m)	1-2 (m)	8-12

Table 3

Interval Training

For those of you who are looking for *more of a challenge*, or generally really enjoy your exercise, then the third option for cardiovascular exercise would be interval training. Interval training is well known for its great benefits on fat burning, and more intense physical exercise in a relatively shorter period of time.

When we step up our efforts to perform interval training, we are no longer working aerobically alone; we begin to train our anaerobic fitness levels as well. Anaerobic means our ability to exercise without the use of oxygen as the main source of fuel. Most of our fuel will come from energy stores within our muscles and body.

Not only does interval training serve as an excellent fat burning tool, but it also develops your cardiovascular fitness levels to a much higher level than the slower, longer duration aerobic cardiovascular training. This is excellent for our health by keeping some of the most important organs in our bodies, such as our heart and lungs, strong and functioning at the highest level.

Many people involved in sports and training for higher intensity activities and events tend to use interval training to maximise their body's ability to cope with the heavier demands placed on their fitness in these disciplines.

When performing an interval training cardiovascular session, you would *begin with a thorough warm up* consisting of dynamic movements as well as slower aerobic cardiovascular exercise for around five to ten minutes to ensure your body is ready for the higher intensity required in this type of training.

Like aerobic intervals you will need two set speeds which you will be working at; one being a moderate speed and one being a high speed. Let's use the treadmill again as an example. The moderate intensity could be 6.0 on the treadmill and the higher working interval could be anything between 7.0 up to around 8.0 or even 9.0.

Work at the slower speed for anywhere between thirty seconds up to two minutes, then increase to the faster level for anywhere between fifteen seconds up to a minute. When starting out, it would be good to use a higher duration of lower speed such as two minutes and a shorter duration of high intensity exercise such as fifteen or twenty seconds.

However, after you've completed a few sessions and begin to improve your fitness level and ability, work to reduce the time spent at the slower speed. This is known as your *recovery interval*. Then increase the duration that you push your body at the higher speed, known as your *work interval*.

One thing I need to make you aware of is the overall nature of this type of cardiovascular exercise. Interval training is a *high intensity activity*, therefore places higher demands and stress on the joints. A long, thorough pre exercise warm up is an *absolute essential,* as well as a proper cool down with a variety of stretches.

However, I do not recommend performing interval training every session that you're in the gym, as this does not give your muscles and joints adequate time to fully recover, adapt and prepare itself for higher intensity work. A good rule is to include an interval training session every once in a while, keeping long steady aerobic exercise as your primary focus.

Perhaps include an interval training session every three to five aerobic cardiovascular sessions. Depending on your physical capabilities and goals from exercise, you may want to perform it more or less often than this.

For others, it may be better not to include this type of training. I don't perform this type of training as the joints at my knee are not particularly strong and have suffered a lot of stress over the years from all my training.

Interval Training Workout Recommendations:

Work Intensity	Rest Intensity	Work Duration	Rest Duration	Total Work Sets
Moderate/high speed	Moderate/low speed	15-30 (s)	1-2 (m)	8-12

Table 4

Other Higher Intensity Cardiovascular Exercise

There are many other forms of high intensive exercise you could incorporate into your exercise routine such as higher intensity interval training, sprints and tabata. However I will not include these as this book is focused on safe, effective exercise that you can include into your routine as a way of life into old age.

Whatever method or type of cardiovascular training that you choose; the most important thing is to make sure you choose something you enjoy or you won't stick with it; if you can look forward to it you will make sure it remains a habit for life. This is the key to your long term adherence and achieving permanent results.

Resistance Exercise

Cardiovascular training, while being the most beneficial to our overall health and fitness levels, is not complete alone. Another form of exercise we need to be aware of and incorporate into our lifestyle is resistance exercise.

Resistance exercise mainly consists of *using our own body weight and the environment around us,* and is an excellent tool for developing physical strength and muscle definition. Resistance exercise builds lean muscle in the areas exercised and the more lean muscle mass we have the leaner we look and the less fat we have.

When I refer to resistance exercise, I'm specifically referring to using your own body weight as the resistance to work against in various movement patterns in order to cause stress on the muscles, tendons and ligaments which force them to grow and repair stronger than their original form.

This greatly benefits the body in handling everyday tasks; further physical activity in the future, reduces the chances of experiencing weakness or injury, and above all creates an excellent appealing well defined, healthy looking physique. I genuinely truly believe that the most important piece of equipment you'll ever have in life for developing natural strength and looking your best is *your very own body.*

Weight training should only be included once you learn and master the key exercises from using your body alone. Using your own body is the most functional way of training and prepares your body to handle the movements and stresses of everyday life. Think of it as building a strong house for yourself; properly lay the foundation with the application of resistance exercises on a frequent basis.

Below I've presented the 20% of key resistance exercises that will bring you 80% of the results in your strength and physique. Squats, press ups and pull ups really are the three most effective resistance exercises.

Once you learn to perform these resistance exercises with perfect technique, and become efficient at them, you can then *progress* the same movement by adding more resistance or even weights to develop your body to higher levels. However right now, let's just focus on the basics and master them in our current routine.

"Where there is no struggle, there is no strength."
– Oprah Winfrey

The 80–20 Resistance Exercises

- **Squats** (Knees should **not** come past your toes, this can be ensured by pushing your bum outwards as you bend your knees as if there is a chair behind you and your going to sit down on it).
- **Press ups** ¾ Press ups, Press ups, Elevated press ups
- **Pull Ups, Assisted Pull-up machine**

- **Tricep dips**
- **Wall squat holds**

When choosing resistance exercises, choose the ones you can perform correctly. If you don't have sufficient strength to perform a particular exercise, try to find another variation that works the same muscle group.

For example pull ups are very difficult for most of us with lower strength levels so consider working the muscles in the back using machines or weights in a specific plane of motion to develop the muscles of our back instead. If you're struggling to perform press ups, consider starting at the ¾ variation and doing what you can until you develop sufficient body awareness and strength to complete some normal press ups.

Start where you are and do what you can. With time and focused practice you will soon be able to progress and perform more repetitions at a greater intensity than what you're currently capable of. Get started, and stay consistent in your efforts until you grow and develop into a much stronger and leaner version of yourself.

Weight Training

Resistance exercises should always be prioritised first and be used to lay the foundation of your muscular training and development. Weight training should been seen as the *secondary chisel* that sharpens the stone and finishes off your physique.

Or *as a progression* to add more resistance to the movement patterns that you have been doing with resistance exercises. For example, once you can do lots of squats with perfect technique using your own body weight and are no longer being challenged because your body as adapted to the pressure, grab two dumbbells from the weight bench in your local gym, hold them by your sides and lower yourself down to perform your squats.

You have now *progressed* your original exercise and will begin to notice a great increase in the strength, function and definition of the muscles in your glutes and thighs. Weight training is the most used form of training for adding lean quality muscle all over our bodies and converting any body fat we have in that area into firm, well defined muscle tissue.

Cardiovascular exercise is great for our health and accelerating weight loss. Resistance training is excellent for building our foundation of body strength and tone. Weight training is the tool for sculpting our bodies and giving us that strong, vibrant athletic look.

Cardio alone will help us lose lots of weight and burn fat; however we often end up just looking like a smaller, scrawny version of our original selves. By really *prioritising resistance and weight training into your routine along with some cardio training,* you will build a strong, athletic, lean looking physique for yourself.

High intensity, controlled weight training is the single most effective tool in burning off body fat and converting it into its lean opposite. The more lean muscle mass you have in your body, the higher your Resting Metabolic Rate, meaning you will burn even more calories naturally while at rest just to maintain this muscle you have gained.

Select a weight that's heavy enough for you to complete around 6 –12 repetitions, while maintaining perfect form at all times. For fat loss and building lean muscle this 6 –12 repetition range would be a good recommendation to work from. This should be *challenging* for you, creating a burning sensation in your muscles, especially as you're doing the final few repetitions of each set.

Aim for around three sets of high intensity weight lifting, pushing your muscles to their current limits. I encourage women as well as men to pick up weights and start pumping iron. By building more muscle you will be torching away body fat; and no, you will not "bulk up" or get "big", contrary to popular belief. You will just become very nicely toned and firm, making you appear sexier and fitter.

One thing to avoid when lifting heavy weights is not to work out the same group of muscles two consecutive days. You must ensure that a minimum of forty-eight hours is allowed for your muscles to recover and grow back stronger.

This is the vital time period where lean muscle gets built and fat slowly diminishes, as long as you feed yourself with the right lean sources of protein, vegetables and drink plenty of water. Do not ruin all your efforts by eating junk food during these muscle recovery hours that follow a heavy weight lifting session.

It is this recovery period where more than ever, *you become what you eat.* Feed yourself only lean, clean, fresh nutritious foods and you're going to come out looking lean, shredded and athletic as a result.

The 80–20 Weight Training Exercises

- **Dumbbell Squats** (By training your leg muscles, the largest muscles in your body, with short, intense workouts (heavier weights, low/moderate reps 4 –12, and little rest time between) you give your body a massive boost of the male sex hormone *testosterone* which will make you feel great, full of energy and vitality and greatly enhances your sex drive, as well as many other health benefits to your body.)
- **Weighted Wall Squat Holds**
- **Dumbbell Shoulder Press**
- **Dumbbell Lateral Raises**
- **Bent Over Dumbbell Lateral Raises**
- **Dumbbell Bicep Curls**
- **Dumbbell Tricep Extensions**
- **Cable Tricep Push Down Machine**
- **Dumbbell Shrugs**

Quality Comes First

The main thing with exercise is *quality*. The quality of the focus, attention and the effort you put into every single movement. Every repetition of every single set, every single time you decide to work out is what counts the most. You have to be *fully present* in the moment; focused on every muscle fibre as you perform each exercise.

Many of us only get out tiny fractions of what we should be because we go *through the motions*. We perform our exercises unconsciously with little or no awareness of what we are actually doing, rushing through each rep and set as quick as we can. This comes from our false belief that ten repetitions are ten repetitions.

Ten press ups for example, are not really ten press ups, when rushed through, only going through half the full range of motion as our minds are occupied elsewhere. We must be there fully with our workouts. **Focus is essential**. Quality always comes first. Two fully conscious, excellent form press ups will contribute towards your results much more than twenty rushed, *half-assed* press ups.

Make sure every rep you perform uses the proper technique while being fully aware of the whole movement in the present moment. This mind-set means you can begin to increase the repetitions and the number of sets. *Quality comes first, then the quantity.* The results will speak for themselves.

Before long you will be looking and feeling strong and sharp. It's all about the *intensity of your focus.* This applies for all types of exercise, whether resistance training, weight training, running your strides on the treadmill or while performing the front crawl strokes in the swimming pool.

Start slowing down while in the gym and really *focus on what you're doing.* Imagine and feel each muscle contracting and relaxing as you perform the exercise through its full range of motion. This will dramatically boost the effectiveness of your exercise sessions and therefore your overall results.

For weight training to be most effective, and give you a permanent athletic looking physique, you should be doing at least two quality weight lifting sessions a week. You need to keep in mind the rule of *"if you don't use it, you lose it."* If you're not continually tearing down your muscles and having them repair themselves as you maintain a high quality diet of lean proteins and vegetables, then your muscles will revert back to their original state.

Make it your goal to schedule two or three training sessions of resistance training, weight training or a mixture of both into your weekly routine. Work out what time of the day feels best for you to get your exercise sessions into your routine. Some people find they are much more energised and in the right frame of mind to train in the morning, while others are much more awake and active during the evenings.

Work with your body clock rather than against it to reap maximum results from your workouts. If your life is very hectic and busy with so many commitments, you may have to get up an hour earlier in order to invest in your health and physique or consider working out from your home. Whatever you decide, schedule your routine.

The more often you train i.e. your exercise *frequency,* and the higher the *intensity,* i.e. your effort level during that exercise, then the greater the *volume* i.e. how much exercise is achieved per session. The higher the volume of exercise: the greater the physical and emotional rewards.

Circuit Training

A great method of training you might enjoy and consider implementing into your routine is circuit training. Circuit training consists of three or more different exercises organised into one workout session, performing one after the other for a set duration of time or number of repetitions on each exercise before moving on to the next one.

The aim is to complete each exercise in sequence before stopping for a brief rest period. This is one set. Perform three to six sets depending on your body's abilities and the amount of time you have to exercise.

Circuit training is the best way to get the most out of your body in the least amount of time. It's also excellent burning fat, adding lean muscle and definition and improving your fitness and general health level. Another benefit of circuit training is that you can do it with others at the gym, your friends or members of your sports club or team which can help to motivate, inspire and add to your enjoyment.

The key, lies in structuring the workout using a combination of anywhere between five and ten different exercises and being fully immersed in the present moment while performing each one with proper technique and your best effort.

Below are a few sample exercises for you to consider incorporating into your circuit training workouts. Of course there are many variations you could use. You can also combine two exercises or more into one single exercise. Such as a dumbbell squat and then shoulder press.

Always remember to *mix things up,* changing what exercises you use each time so you're never repeating the same exact workout over and over again. *Variety* stimulates your body to continue to grow and adapt as it is constantly being stimulated by new stresses and therefore works different muscles and body parts around your body.

Exercises to choose from when designing your circuit:

Upper Body:

Press up variations	Dumbbell/barbell bicep curls	Pull up variations	Dumbbell/barbell shrugs
Dumbbell/barbell bench press	Tricep bench dips	Dumbbell shoulder variations	Dumbbell hammer curls
Dumbbell/barbell shoulder press	Dumbbell/ barbell tricep extensions	Dumbbell/barbell bent over rows	Dumbbell shoulder arms out hold

Table 5

Abdominals and Core:

Sit up variations	Crunch variations	Plank variations
Lower leg raise variations	Back extension variations	Oblique heel touches
Russian Twist Variations	Medicine ball abdominal exercise variations	Abdominal Rollout variations

Table 6

Lower Body:

Bodyweight squats	Lunges	Step up variations
Wall squats	Leg press machines	Walking lunges
Dumbbell/ barbell squats	Dumbbell/barbell lunges	Lateral lunges

Table 7

Cardiovascular:

Star jumps	Burpees	Running on the spot
Skipping rope	Cone runs/sprints	Box jumps
Step ups	Frog jumps	Battle rope waves and alpha bag slams

Table 8

When scheduling your circuit workout, make it your goal to include three to six full rounds of anywhere between three and twelve different types of exercises. Create a set time to perform each exercise of between ten and thirty seconds, depending on factors such as your current fitness level, your goals and the ability of the other members of your group.

Circuit Training Exercise Recommendations:

Duration to perform each exercise	Sets to perform of whole circuit	Rest period between each set of circuit
15 – 30s	3 – 5 sets	30s – 2m

Table 9

The photo here shows a basic, six-station exercise circuit to give you an idea of the layout and structure when creating your own circuit. In the photos that follow I

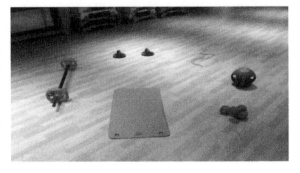

71

give you one of the most effective uses you can make of your time while in the gym for gaining lean muscle, burning body fat, increasing your strength, fitness and health levels. It's an all-time favourite mini-circuit of mine and the clients that I trained while I was a personal trainer.

Simple, only three exercises, yet very powerful for achieving great results as it includes the three basic human movement patterns, (squatting, pulling and pushing). The repetition range I recommend for you in the chart below has also been well designed with the correct number of repetitions to perform of each exercise in order to create an even muscular balance in your chest, lower body and back. This will prevent any unattractive muscular imbalances occurring and is designed to reduce the potential for injury.

An example of creating an imbalance would be to do hundreds of press ups, and no upper back work in order to balance the front and back parts of your upper body evenly. For example, if you were to do only press ups, over time the alignment of your body would become curved due to having too much muscle weight on your chest in relation to your upper back. So make sure to keep the repetitions in the range that I have recommended to you in in Table 10.

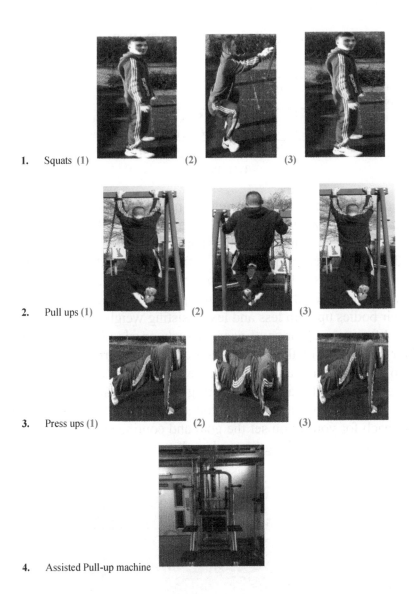

1.   Squats (1)   (2)   (3)

2.   Pull ups (1)   (2)   (3)

3.   Press ups (1)   (2)   (3)

4.   Assisted Pull-up machine

Exercise Recommendations for the Squat, Pull, Press Workout:

Exercise	Reps		Sets of Circuit	Rest Between Sets
Squats (Bodyweight or Weighted)	10 – 20			
Pull ups (Or assisted machine)	3 – 6			
Press ups	10 – 20		3 – 6	30s – 2m

Table 10

If you do not have enough strength to perform a pull up, *consider using an assisted pull up machine* at your local gym if available. The great majority of my clients, particularly the women and underdeveloped men, did not have sufficient strength to perform a proper pull up when I first started to work with them. However over time, with the use of the assisted pull up machine, they were able to pull their bodies up with less and less assisting weight.

After a month or so of *progressively overloading* the muscles in their back most of them were then able to perform a full proper pull up without any assistance. Some even went on to complete multiple pull ups. It's all about starting where you are and focusing on tiny little improvements over a longer period of time. Nothing is out of reach for you if you set the goal and continue to work towards it every time you're in the gym, each and every week.

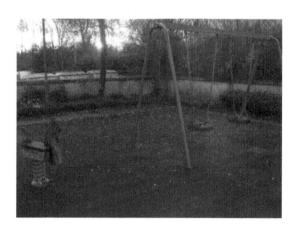

If your local gym does not have an assisted pull up machine then substitute this exercise for another exercise that works the muscles located in your upper back, such as dumbbell or barbell upright or bent-over rows. Or even use another fixed machine that develops your upper back such as the lat pull down or seated row machine.

The picture above shows the gym that I use to perform the majority of my exercise. The swing park outside my flat. Squats, pull ups and press ups are a few of the most rewarding exercises you could possibly perform to building your physique and developing physical strength. There is absolutely no excuse not to exercise, if you cannot afford a gym membership or are pressed for time, then get outside into your back yard and get a work out session in.

Abdominal and Core Exercise

For as little as five to ten minutes a day, a few days a week, you could develop a hard, firm midsection that links your upper and lower body together and creates a strong foundation of support for your body to work from. Not only that, but if you have been adhering to the principles I have taught you on nutrition earlier, as part of your habitual way of living, you should have achieved a reasonably low level of body fat which will enable your six pack set of abdominal muscles to shine brightly through.

Training the muscles of your core is a very important aspect of your physical fitness and supports all the internal organs and structures of your body. As we age our stomach muscles are often neglected, which causes them to weaken and often leaves us carrying around a *spare bag* wherever we go. This bag is something most of us would rather not leave the house with; after all why carry something around with you all day that serves no good purpose?

As I mentioned earlier, your eating habits are the main determinant of the size and type of bag that you take around with you. However, the part of the equation that hardens, and shapes this bag into a more appealing design is exercise. There are hundreds of different variations of controlled movements you can perform to target those abdominal muscles in your midsection and cause them to tighten and harden up. However, I like to keep things simple, and will just give you one workout that you can use to work your entire core as much as you would like, hitting all the main muscle groups: front, back and the sides of your midsection. Below are the exercises you will need and the order in which to perform them.

Complete one set of either ten, twelve, fifteen, or twenty repetitions of each exercise, finished with a plank isometric hold for as long as you can until you reach failure. The number of repetitions you perform on each abdominal exercise will depend on your current ability and core strength. However as you begin to incorporate this abdominal circuit into your routine, you will be able to increase the repetitions and duration you can hold your plank before you collapse to the floor.

After you complete the set amount of repetitions for each exercise and your plank hold until you fail, you need to take a short rest period of anywhere between ten to thirty seconds. This rest period must be very brief, in order to keep your abdominals stimulated to create a high enough level of stress to strengthen them. As for the number of sets needed for the full benefit, a minimum of three to six sets are required depending on your current level and ability. The main point I want to emphasise again is: always work from a focused mind-set. Focus and concentration in the present moment, on the area of your core being worked, is the key to getting results in this workout.

Visualise the muscle group that you're working and perform every repetition in a slow and controlled manner. Imagine the muscle fibres being torn and squeezed as you go through the movement of each rep. When your muscles start to burn, notice that this is a sign of progress. Every repetition you complete while your abdominals are burning, without giving up or quitting will be contributing to the overall results and effectiveness of the session. You want to feel the burn and continue pushing out more repetitions anyway. Learn to enjoy this burning sensation as it is part of process and directly affects the results you will achieve. No pain, no gain.

Core Training Exercises

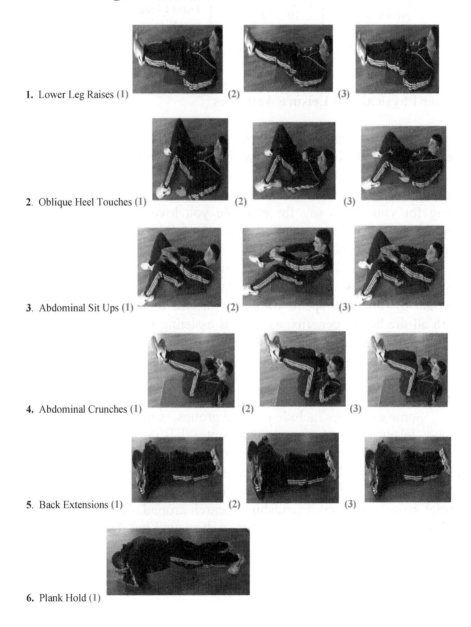

1. Lower Leg Raises **(1)** **(2)** **(3)**

2. Oblique Heel Touches **(1)** **(2)** **(3)**

3. Abdominal Sit Ups **(1)** **(2)** **(3)**

4. Abdominal Crunches **(1)** **(2)** **(3)**

5. Back Extensions **(1)** **(2)** **(3)**

6. Plank Hold **(1)**

Exercise	Reps
Lower Leg Raises	10-20
Oblique Heel Touches	10 – 20 each side
Abdominal Sit ups	10 – 20
Abdominal Crunches	10 – 20
Back Extensions	10 – 20

Total Circuit Sets	Rest between each set
3-6	10-30s

Table 11

Other Physical and Leisure Activities

For many of us reading this book, taking a run or signing up to a health club and lifting weights may be too physically demanding. Or we may simply not have the passion or the interest. This is absolutely fine but is *not an excuse* not to exercise. It's about finding the right thing for you. Let's say for example you love walking. You can support your weight loss efforts by scheduling a few long walks throughout the week.

Although walking tends to burn a low number of calories compared to going for a run or swim, by increasing the distance or amount of time you spend walking you will be providing yourself with all the health benefits, as well as assisting weight and body fat loss. The goal is always to make sure you find physical activity that you can *enjoy*. Today, if you look and ask around your community, you will find all sorts of leisure activities and clubs that you can become a part of.

Some examples include running groups, walking groups, sports clubs, leisure events, community centre leisure activities, health clubs, community gyms, swimming pools, community fitness classes, outdoor boot camps, personal training, rowing clubs, athletics, yoga and dancing classes etc. You might also enjoy the social aspects and new friendships. Search around, do your research online and in your local newspaper. Ask around but don't shy away from exercise!

Get Active

Include movement throughout the day as much as possible. Think of how you can incorporate light exercise and activity into your daily routine as healthier lifestyle choices. For example, during the summer months get your bike out of the shed and cycle to and from work. Go on bike and picnic trips at the weekend with your family. Decide to hike a large hill or small mountain as a personal challenge. Start attending the circuit training classes at your local community centre or gym.

Walk to work. Walk to the shops and go for regular walks with your spouse, dog or whole family. Consider building your own gym or workout area in your home or garage; somewhere for you to go to a few times a week. Exercise should always be a *lifestyle.* When you go on holidays, consider trying out the gyms, go for a run along the beach, and spend time swimming in the sea. Consider buying and enrolling in a fitness DVD training program and get exercising right now in your own living room.

Live actively by reducing the time you spend sitting. Get moving. If you're considering attending the fitness classes regularly, I cannot emphasise the value that you will gain in your fitness, health and physique from attending them consistently. You do not need to be excellent or even fit to join. *Just show up and participate,* even if that means you will be spending half the workout sitting by the side of the class gasping for air and gulping down water, taking short breaks. The class instructors are trained understanding people who are quite used to new members.

They only expect you to do your best. They will encourage your progress as you continue to attend their classes. After just a few weeks of getting into a regular routine of classes, you're going to notice the difference. When I was a personal trainer I walked around the gym facility, initiated conversations with newer members and encouraged them to come along to all my classes. Despite their initial doubt, a few weeks later every one of those who came were in great physical shape and were enjoying the classes so much that they couldn't afford to miss a single session. Their health, physiques and their quality of life had dramatically improved just from taking that *first step*. Give it a try for yourself; *you have nothing to lose and plenty to gain*. Book yourself in to the next upcoming class down at the gym and *just do what you can.* Everyone starts somewhere.

> *"The harder I work, the luckier I get."*
> **– Gary Player**

Post Workout Stretches and Attention

Another essential, just like the pre exercise warm up movements and preparation, is the care and attention you give your muscles and body *after* you complete any strenuous physical activity. The predominant muscle groups involved in the exercise must be stretched out and shaken off if you want to maintain your flexibility and prevent stiffness, pain and injury in the future. After exercising and working your muscles you will have created a lot of tension within them and if you do not take the time to stretch and loosen them, you may begin to feel more fatigued. To release this build-up of energy, muscles need to be stretched. There are two main types of stretches.

Static stretches are used to ensure we *maintain* our original flexibility levels after creating tension within that muscle through resistance and exertion. To perform a static stretch, we would have to hold our muscle in a fixed position that causes that muscle to increase slightly in length and then keep it held in this position for anywhere between fifteen and thirty seconds.

Developmental stretches are one step further in that they work to *improve* our current level of flexibility at the joint and muscle targeted. Just like static stretches, we will be increasing the length of the muscle and holding it in place without any movement. However we need to aim to hold this for a minimum of thirty seconds, up to around two minutes. Every thirty seconds, we slightly increase the length of the stretch by a tiny amount; therefore lengthening the muscle. The one rule that is essential before you stretch any of your muscles, in a static or developmental manner, is that your muscles must be warm and your mind should be in a calm, relaxed state.

Never hold or force a stretch on a cold muscle or you will be at risk of creating a small tear that can result in severe pain or injury. Also, you need to put yourself into a *relaxed state of mind.* There are many ways to relax while stretching. You could use calm, chilled out music, a long relaxing warm bath, or even the exhaustion and fatigue that results from a good workout session is all you need.

I highly recommend that you take the time after every workout session and even schedule single, separate sessions devoted entirely to stretching alone. This is essential if you want to promote super high levels of energy and vitality, while feeling young, light and fresh, and preventing any possibility of injuries in the future.

Below is a sample full body stretch workout that I often perform during a single session after a nice warm bath in order to keep myself injury free and flexible. When performed correctly, fully focused on every stretch, you will feel great afterwards.

1. **Calf stretch** (30 seconds – 1 minute relaxed hold on each calve.
2. **Seated floor hamstring stretch** (30 seconds – 1 minute relaxed hold on each hamstring)
3. **Lying prone quadriceps stretch** (30 seconds – 1 minute relaxed hold on each quadricep)
4. **Prone cobra lower back and abdominal stretch** (30 seconds – 1 minute relaxed hold)
5. **Cat stretch** (lower back) – (30 seconds – 1 minute relaxed hold).
6. **Hip flexor lunge stretch** (30 seconds – 1 minute relaxed hold each hip flexor)
7. **Lying straight-leg hamstring stretch using a towel** (30 seconds – 1 minute relaxed hold each hamstring)
8. **Lower back stretch and mobility** – rocking knees to chest, then rocking side to side – (10 knees to chest, 5 rocks each side. Repeat 3 times).

9. **More stretches** (optional) – Deltoids, Triceps, Upper back, Trapezius, Biceps, Pectorals, Adductors, and any other muscle groups of your own choice.

There are many types of static and developmental stretches that you can incorporate into your routine. If you find that your muscles are very stiff and tight as a result of your regular intensive training routines, consider investing in a foam roller in order to roll over the rough spots you may have in the muscles to produce a similar effect to a hard, body massage. This will help to loosen your muscles up, release trapped stored energy and improve your muscles' flexibility and recovery from exercise.

"Movement is a medicine for creating change in a person's physical, emotional and mental states."
– Carol Welch

Summary:

• Always begin all of your exercise sessions with a thorough 5 –10 minute warm up consisting of light cardiovascular exercise with full body, dynamic movement stretches.

• Schedule a minimum of one resistance training exercise session into your weekly routine and push your muscles to their limits in order to cause them to grow back stronger, helping you develop and forge out a lean looking physical appearance. Your resistance training session could involve resistance exercises, weight lifting, a circuit training session or even a combination of each.

• Schedule a minimum of one cardiovascular exercise session into your weekly routine lasting a minimum of 15 – 30 minutes of long steady aerobic exercise to improve your physical and mental health and wellbeing as well as stimulating weight and fat loss.

- Perform the abdominal circuit workout a minimum of two days throughout your weekly routine and push your abdominal muscles past the burn they experience to strengthen and tone up your midsection.

- Consider how you can incorporate more physical activity or movement into your current weekly routine in order to improve your health and wellbeing. This could include walking to work, going for a family bike trip at the weekend, doing the gardening more often or any other active ideas that you can come up with.

- Always finish off your exercise sessions with a thorough 5 – 10 minute cool down consisting of static or developmental stretch holds on all the major muscle groups used during your exercise session.

-5-

The Power of Planning

Plan to Live an Active Lifestyle

Reading this book may change your mind-set and improve your habits. But reading alone will never produce results and improvements in how you look, feel and the overall quality of your life. You must take action. Yet, even action alone is not enough. Action without thinking is said to be the greatest cause of failure. It is also said that for every minute you spend planning, you save hours, days, weeks and years in the long term.

For example, planning your month in advance may require you to spend around ten minutes of your time with a cup of tea and a pen and paper engaging in a period of focused thinking. However, once you have scheduled how you'll spend your time, all you need to do each day is invest your energies in those goals. Take the shopping list as a simple example for focusing your time productively. When you write out what you need to buy in advance, you waste little time at the supermarket, you get what you need and get out again.

Consider your work day. Many top performing employees and managers take a few minutes the night before or in the morning of their working day to prioritise and plan. This means their day is focused on those key tasks. It is said that "if you fail to plan, you plan to fail".

While no plan is perfect, it is clearly better than no plan at all.

In this chapter I'll show you a powerful method of planning out your exercise sessions up to a month in advance and how it keeps you focused and in control of your time, health, and life. It only requires you invest as little as five minutes at the beginning of the month.

> *"Planning is bringing the future into the present so that you can do something about it now."*
> **– Alan Lakein**

Your Two Tools

There are two tools that can maximise your planning and your actions that I will discuss in this chapter. But first of all remember that you need to be accountable. If you make the plan, ensure you see it through. This is aided by the support of those around you. The Law of Cause and Effect says that if we do it, we get a result.

The Law of Compensation says that we must give first before we can receive. We will get back exactly what we give out of ourselves. The more effort and time that we spend on our health and fitness, the more we will be paid back in terms of long-term health benefits. The really successful people in any area of life take this Universal Law one step further and apply the Law of Overcompensation.

This law states that success comes to those who always put in more than they take out. They find a way to schedule extra physical exercise and activity into their lives, ensure that they are always doing more exercise this week than they did last week and of a higher quality of intensity and focus. To improve and get higher and better results, you must put more into what you're currently doing. It's quite simple, yet overlooked because as humans, we are programmed to do less than we're capable of and to seek comfort over challenge.

Combining the Law of Cause and Effect with the Law of Overcompensation to your nutrition and physical activity means you put yourself in full control of the results you achieve. No excuses. It's all on you.

"If you fail to plan, you are planning to fail."
– Benjamin Franklin

Tool One: Monthly Calendar

Take five to ten minutes at the end of every month to plan the following month's exercise and physical activities. Plan the type of exercise you will be performing each day, but I also want you to set monthly goals and targets to strive to achieve in both your exercise and your life.

Once you have created your plan at the beginning of the month, try not to think about it or analyse it. Instead, focus all your energies on living your life and getting your exercise sessions completed, using pens to mark off each exercise or activity session after completion at the end of your day before you retire for the night. By following through on all your scheduled exercise commitments, you will experience a great sense of control.

Continue completing each session without missing any of them out and you will generate a feeling of momentum. If, however, something happens and you need to miss out a session, don't beat yourself up. Tell yourself that's okay. Some things in your life will have to come first but now you need to fit in what you missed another time; whether the following day, or later on that week. Simply add that missed exercise session into your calendar the next day or as soon as possible and get it done.

Never skip a session that you need as the only person you will be cheating is yourself. If you cannot trust and rely on yourself, then you will never be successful in achieving your goals in life. Nobody can do it for you. At the end of each day when you're back at home, you need to check off the exercise and activities that you completed on your calendar. This should be a daily habit.

You may choose to use multi coloured pens to mark off each type of exercise session or activity as I do myself. For example, you could put a red tick by each resistance or weight training session and a blue tick by each cardiovascular training session. I find that by doing this it's easier to tally up all my sessions and activities at the end of the month.

"Nothing is particularly hard if you divide it into small jobs."
– Henry Ford

The photos here are an example of my month of exercise planned in advance as well as roughly what your calendar should look like at the end of the month once you adhere to all of your commitments.

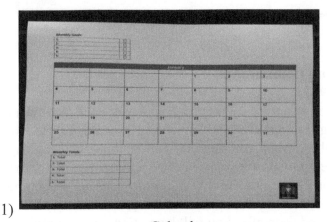

1)

Calendar

2)

Planned

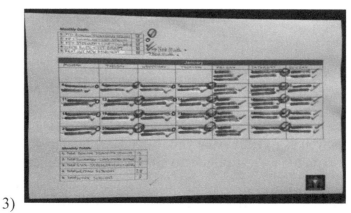

3)

Completed

Planning and Committing

Write out your exercise routine for each week once, and then commit to following through every session fully. No excuses. Be where you said you will be when you said you will be there, even on days when you don't feel like it. *Act your way into feeling.* Get out of the house, put one foot in front of the other and the very act of getting to the right place at the right time and starting off slowly will generate momentum and soon after you will be getting on as normal.

Sometimes professional athletes don't really feel like hitting the gym, however they are **committed.** They will be there, put their heads down and do what they know they should do, whether they feel like it in that moment or not. And so must you. Make a full personal commitment. In the beginning you may have to call upon and use your willpower and personal discipline. However if you just get started and stay focused, you will soon turn your planned exercise routine into a *habit* and it will not require as much energy for you to start and complete all your workouts.

Focus on completing the scheduled exercise sessions you have created for yourself just one day, one workout at a time. Don't overwhelm yourself with the big picture. Master the present moments in your life; get into the habit of making each day successful, one at a time. By always completing your exercise session each scheduled day, they will soon begin to accumulate and add up. When you follow through and complete seven days doing the exercise that you scheduled for yourself, you will have had a successful week. Four successful weeks, completing and scoring off all your exercise will result in a successful month. Twelve successful months will be a successful year.

Continue to produce successful years of exercise and activity from here onwards and you will have a long, lean and healthy successful life that you can be proud of. The key is not to become overwhelmed with the big picture, just focus on the twenty-four hour day that you have ahead of you. Before long you will wake up one morning, take a look at yourself and realise just how far you have come.

Reviewing, Analysing and Adjusting

At the end of every month, you must schedule five or ten minutes to review your calendar. First, you want to add up all your sessions in each type of exercise, cardio, resistance and so on. Check if you met your goals and targets for each one. If you have, then great you are on track and are exercising great character and discipline in your life. If not, you must decide if you're really serious about getting into excellent shape and how bad you truly want it.

Look back over your month overall. Decide what activities you may need to do more of next month in order to achieve better results. Decide if there are any activities that you may be doing and getting very little in return and remove these unproductive activities. You will have learned a lot about yourself, what works for you, what doesn't work, how your body responds to specific exercise and routines when you do this.

Now, use all this wisdom you have gained to write out your weekly routine into your calendar for the following month. Decide if you're going to increase your sessions or change your routine. Check off any personal goals you achieved. Set yourself higher or new goals for the following month. Take the time to write out your following month's routine in terms of exercise and physical activity in advance. Then put the calendar back in its place and get busy in action and manifesting your goals and desires into reality.

> *"It is common sense to take a method and try it.*
> *If it fails, admit it frankly and try another.*
> *But above all, try something."*
> **– Franklin D. Roosevelt**

Download Your Calendar

You can buy your own yearly calendar from places like the local newsagents or I can offer you a way to download one. Use it for planning and tracking your exercise and activity. Keep it in your bedroom, office or pin it to your fridge. Put it up somewhere in your house that you will pass it each evening at the end of your day in order to score off your exercise at the end of each day. You can download a free, monthly exercise calendar from my website at: www.momentumpersonaldevelopment.co.uk Print out the twelve months and keep them together. You can use this same template year after year free of charge.

Monthly Goal Setting

I cannot emphasise the value and process of *continual goal setting throughout your life.* The majority of us grow old and lose a sense of challenge and purpose in our lives after we graduate from school and get a job. Working from nine to five and living for the weekend with no personal targets and accomplishments we truly desire can be soul-destroying. So set goals.

These goals can be anything, such as completing a further education course in your field to upgrade your knowledge and value at work, to getting a date with the pretty single girl you're attracted to in your town, getting a pay rise or promotion at your work from increasing your contribution and efforts to the company, or saving up a specific amount of money to put towards your yearly holiday.

Whatever the goals you decide to choose and focus on, the key is to *select a few that you truly desire.* Having a few goals usually works better than having too many. You only have so much time so the objective is to focus your attention on a few things that you can achieve. It's better to set and achieve two well-defined goals each month, than fail to achieve a list of ten impossible goals.

Choose one thing; fully focus your efforts each and every day working towards its attainment, chipping away at it like chopping down a tree, until you finally receive the result you desire. Celebrate and acknowledge your accomplishment, then refocus your attention and efforts on the next goal. Make good use of your calendar by setting a few, empowering goals that you truly want to achieve for yourself or someone else in your life.

Don't worry about whether or not you achieve it at the end of the month, as some goals take much longer to achieve. As long as you take some kind of daily action, big or small, eventually you will crack the code and make it a reality. For all goals that you don't achieve by the end of your month, as you review and analyse your efforts, simply *carry them over to the following month.*

Goals can serve as a very powerful source of motivation towards your exercise efforts. Any important upcoming events in your life such as a friend or family member's wedding, an upcoming holiday, a weekend away, going on a date, or other events where it would be great for you to look and feel at your very best should be written down under the date on your calendar.

Now with this date down, you can begin to *work backwards* and plan all your daily exercise sessions and fuel them with renewed motivation and focus. You're also much more likely to enjoy the process when you know exactly why you're doing it. You can take things a bit further by setting more challenging goals such as marathons, half marathons, tough mudder events, local runs, sporting events and so on.

This gives you an end goal that you can use to challenge yourself in all your workouts and efforts up until the day of your event or challenge.

"Practice yourself in little things, and thence proceed to greater."
– Epictetus

Tool Two: Exercise Accountability Diary

A diary is a *great accountability tool and personal motivator.* Once you have completed your day's exercise and you're back at the house take a minute to log what you did in terms of exercise for that day. Include all the details such as the weight you lifted, the reps, the sets, the different exercises, the duration of cardiovascular exercise, and your stretches and so on.

This works as a great tool for measuring your progress and development, as you will be able to look back over the previous months and use that as a reference. It will help you decide if you need to step up the efforts that you're putting into your workouts, as well as make it easier to keep you on track with staying consistent in your activity levels. For example, you will know if you're *off track* when you start to log too many consecutive "REST" days in a row.

One of the best ways to make sure you adhere to your exercise schedule and put in great quality workouts every single time is to *learn to love it.* Learn to love your training. Choose the types and methods of exercises that you enjoy doing the most. Learn to love the improvements in mental, emotional and physical wellbeing that come as a result of pushing yourself with each exercise session that you complete. Think about the consequences of missing a workout and how it will negatively affect your physical, mental, emotional and spiritual wellbeing. By working hard and completing your workouts in your

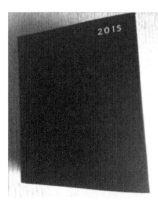

exercise routine each and every week, the positive effects will spill out into all the other areas of your life. You'll feel happier, more positive, energetic, and in control of yourself. Everyone around you will benefit.

Applying the Principle of Progressive Overload

Once you have your schedule of cardiovascular, resistance, weight training, sports, and physical leisure activities written down on your calendar and you're taking action on a daily basis, recording your efforts on your diary, you're now heading in the right direction to becoming the strongest, fittest, leanest and healthiest person that you can be.

However, repeating the same routines over and over, you may notice that your body and health are not developing the way that you would like them to and you seem stuck at a certain level. You cannot get lower than a certain weight, reduce your body fat below a particular percentage or look as defined as you visualise yourself to be. This brings us to what we call the **Principle of Insanity** (discussed in more detail later).

This principle basically says that when you *keep doing the same things over and over again, you will only get the same results that you have always got.* Therefore, we need to do something more; something different to our normal current routine. We need to *progress our efforts,* either by doing more exercise sessions, increasing the amount of time and exercise we put into each session, pushing ourselves harder by lifting heavier weights or running a little faster.

This is known as *Progressive Overload.* Progressive overload is the idea that once we perform a certain exercise, activity, or routine a few times, our body will have grown *accustomed* to the stress that we place on it from this activity. Therefore the only way to create further change and development in that part of our body or fitness is to push ourselves a little bit harder than we did before.

We need to systematically increase the duration of our cardiovascular sessions, the weight that we lift and the amount of times we train each week gradually as time goes on and we get used to our current routines. Never go backwards. Always look for ways to increase your overall weekly and monthly workload. However don't rush things.

By trying to increase your outputs in each area of your exercise routines too soon you could cause injury, burnout or take away any enjoyment and fun that you experience from the exercise experience itself. Your body needs a few weeks or months to grow stronger through all the stresses you are placing on it therefore make sure that you *systematically* increase your exercise duration, intensity and frequency only a *small amount* every few weeks.

An example of how I apply progressive overload to my own exercise routine is my long steady distance cardiovascular sessions. Every fortnight I increase the speed of the treadmill by a tiny fraction of about 0.2. For example: I do a light jog for thirty minutes at 6.0 twice a week, for two weeks. This would be four sessions over the two week period. I would then increase the speed to 6.2 and repeat the process for another two weeks, or four sessions.

Then after these two weeks are up, I would increase the speed to 6.3 or 6.4. The increases should be nothing dramatic. Only increase your exercise by very small fractions over a longer period of time. By doing this, you ensure that your body can improve in a safe and progressive manner and it eliminates the chance of you experiencing injury or losing enthusiasm in your training.

You have got to *think long term.* 0.2 may be nothing in just two weeks, but if you were to increase by 1.0 every two weeks, would your body be able to cope with the increase twelve months from now?18.0 speed for thirty minutes on the treadmill? I don't think so. I don't even think the machine is programmed that high. Small changes systematically incorporated or a long period of time will pay off in your physique, health and fitness levels and your body will naturally adapt to cope with the demands placed upon it.

Nothing is better than the feeling and knowing that you're making progress no matter how small. As long as each and every month you're moving upwards with your efforts and putting in just a little bit more each time, you will feel great about yourself, and your body will never be stuck at a plateau where you can no longer see and feel small changes taking place.

See the picture that follows as an example of my own logged daily workouts:

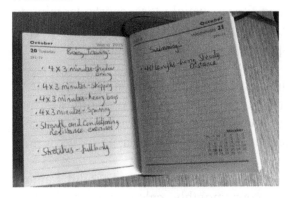

Plan Your Work and Work Your Plan

The biggest cause of failure in achieving your weight loss, fat loss, health, fitness and physique goals will come from failure to stick to your scheduled exercise plan and improved eating habits. This is why making good use of this yearly calendar in setting, monitoring and achieving your life and fitness goals will hold yourself accountable and ensure that you achieve your desires.

Action is the key to getting what you want in life. **And you can get it.**

> *"Self-discipline is the ability to make yourself do what you should do, when you should do it, whether you feel like it or not."*
> **– Elbert Hubbard**

Summary:

- Download your free monthly goal and exercise schedule planner from momentumpersonaldevelopment.co.uk or take a trip to your local newsagents to buy a monthly calendar for this year.

- Write down your current life goals that you want to achieve for yourself in any area of your life, whether it's family, relationships, income, career, health and fitness, weight loss, sports, learning to play a new instrument, learning a new skill, reading a specific number of books on a specific topic or any other goals

- Schedule all your cardio sessions into your monthly calendar to put you into that slight negative energy balance in order to lose weight, strip off body fat. Increase your cardiovascular fitness and improve your overall health and wellbeing levels.

- Schedule all your resistance, weight training and circuit training individual sessions into your monthly calendar to build lean muscle tissue, burn away body fat and sculpt your body into a very attractive, athletic, healthy looking figure.

- Schedule all your sport, fitness classes, leisure activities or commitments that you're already a part of, or would like to try out to see if you enjoy them. These are activities you could make a positive habit in your current routine and incorporate into your monthly calendar to contribute towards your weight loss, physique, enjoyment, social life and overall health and wellbeing.

- Total up all your scheduled sessions for each type of exercise or physical activity choice and write down your monthly goals for each type of activity. This allows you to review them at the end of your month and see if you have adhered to your plan. If not, you can decide if you would like to make any changes for next month's target of sessions, based on your time schedule, results and own personal satisfaction.

- Once you have completed your monthly plan and targets for your goals, exercise and activities for the month, put your calendar away somewhere that you will see at the end of every single day where you can check off your daily exercise and activities once you have completed them. Now, all you have to do is get busy living and working on your goals, staying consistent in your efforts and making sure that you invest your time on those activities that will give you the highest return for your efforts.

-6-

Mind-Set

Everything Starts in the Mind

Desire is a sense of longing or hoping for an outcome. We feel it in our heart, we see it in our mind; we think it, we imagine it, we want it. Desire is the *requirement* needed to start the process, and it's what will motivate us to change. We want it but we have to keep working at it to achieve it.

There is a natural tendency for is us to revert back to old, comfortable, habits so *our mind* must be stronger than our body to maintain this new improved way of living. Most of us focus on the external, what we can see and do. However *the internal* is the most important part in order to create and maintain lasting results in the external world. Before we can do anything, we must first think of it and see it clearly in our mind's eye. We need to support our physical efforts in the best ways by seeing the slimmest, trimmest, healthiest version of ourselves.

Why do *you* want to lose weight? This will be your ultimate motivating factor. The single most important determinant of progress is the *intensity of your desire*. Are you sick and tired of being overweight?

What is required of you to succeed are a handful of daily behavioural changes and a shift in mind-set. The mind and body are not separate. By putting your focus on developing your body with the right foods, liquids, sensible consistent exercise, adequate sleep and relaxation, your mind will benefit. The body directly influences the brain. For example, think back to a time when you may have felt stressed or anxious and then taken a long walk or engaged in some light consistent exercise only to feel calm, content and relaxed afterwards.

We must work to develop both our body and our minds simultaneously. The outward expression of our physical body is influenced by our current state of mind. By making sure we're always feeding our minds with positive inspirational, motivational and educational life-affirming materials through good books, audio CDs and other positive like-minded people, we are taking control of our own physiology. We are directly improving our attitudes, actions and the quality of results that we will ultimately achieve.

Pushing out extra repetitions and taking your body well past your comfort zone into places that it has never been will allow it to grow stronger and leaner than it's even been. You really have to *be there* and focus *in the moment* using your mind in order to stimulate maximum results. In this chapter I will share with you some ideas that may open up your current ways of thinking to help you see things from new perspectives. Once understood these will make achieving your goals and getting through harder times in your life a lot more manageable and easier to accomplish. The power of the mind is unmatched. Take control and build up your mental muscles and they will be the fuel behind all physical efforts and activities in your life.

"Reality is wrong. Dreams are for real."
– Tupac Shakur

Feed the Positive and Starve the Negative

One of the number one factors, and probably the single most effective indicator, of one's health is a *positive mental attitude.* While this might not come naturally, you can work to develop it. By keeping your thoughts on positive things rather than negative things, you will soon bring about positive change. So be aware of who and what is around you that is influencing your thinking.

While some things are not in our control, *many things are.* We can't control where we are born, what start we get in life for example, however *we can choose* who we spend our time with. *We can choose* how we feed our mind through what we decide to watch, read, listen to and believe in. We can all be positive and negative to varying degrees but for a positive life we should try to spend less time with the people who are predominantly negative; the ones who criticise, belittle, crush our dreams and hopes and drain our energy.

Instead we should spend most of our time around people who nourish us, lift us up and love and accept us unconditionally. Similarly we can start replacing the time we spend on unproductive, negative activities with more positive, supportive choices that build character and spirit and move us towards our goals. Swap newspapers and magazines for positive inspirational, educational and motivational books.

Only watch TV with a purpose for example that educates, relaxes and entertains. Listen to more positive, clean, uplifting and inspiring music rather than songs that make you feel blue, down or vulgar. Join groups and clubs in your community to meet like-minded positive people. Continually put yourself into a positive environment that's conductive to your development as a person and the goals you want to achieve.

Keep feeding your mind with positive information to raise your energy level, attitude and positive outlook. This is all a *choice* that you can make each and every day. You can *choose* to sink with the negative or rise with the positive.

"Don't wish it were easier, wish you were better."
                                                        – Jim Rohn

People who are generally more negative will only drain your energy; distract you from making progress towards being the best person you can be in your life and achieving the things that you truly want for yourself. So if you can, love them but choose to spend less time with them.

As you find happiness and success there will always be someone who wants to squash that achievement, to tell you that something cannot be done. Others may feel left out or even jealous once you begin to make changes and see the results. Most of the time these responses are *unconscious*, so accept this, never dislike or put down another person for this. Understand how they may be feeling or thinking. Realise that their mind-set may be completely different to yours and they do not understand your motivation. Love them unconditionally but don't allow them or their expectations to deter you from your goal.

As you begin to make changes in your life as a result of the information provided in this book and begin to think and act differently in more positive, constructive, successful ways, you'll notice that you no longer resonate or 'click' with certain people in your life. The reason for this is that your brain chemistry has altered and you may no longer be on the same wavelength because you have consciously chosen to grow and change. But by letting go of the old, you are creating more room in your life to allow the new to come into it.

"Be careful the environment you choose for it will shape you; be careful the friends you choose for you will become like them."
– W. Clement Stone

Positive Mind-set Strategies you may want to implement:

1. Get in Control

Accept full and complete responsibility for everything you are, everything you have and everything you will become in life. No excuses. By taking responsibility you put yourself in control of your life and release any build-up of negative energy that is holding you back. Decide to forgive everyone and everything from your past and focus fully on what and where you want your life to be in the future.

Then get busy today, living fully in the present moment, taking action towards what you want to be, doing and having in your life. Accepting full, complete responsibility at all times is the key to gaining control over your life and attitude. You cannot change what happens to you in life, but you can always change *how you respond* to what happens to you.

A basic rule in human psychology is the Law of Control. This law states that as humans, we all feel positive about ourselves *to the degree* that we feel we are in control of our lives. Similarly we will feel negative about ourselves *to the degree* that we feel that we are *not* in control of our lives. Your job is to take control. Make use of your monthly exercise calendar, set true goals for yourself that you deeply believe are possible for you to achieve, plan all your meals ahead of time, organise your kitchen the way you want your body to look and so on.

Do whatever it takes to gain as much control in each area of your life so that things flow naturally in the direction you want them to. The more control you take in your choices and actions, the less the external environment will dictate your body weight, amount of body fat and overall quality of health.

In Personality Psychology, *locus of control* refers to the extent to which an individual believes that they are in control of the events affecting them. A person's "locus" (Latin for "place" or "location") of control can either be internal or external depending on the extent that a person believes they can control the outcomes of the events that occur in their lives. Individuals who have a strong internal locus of control believe that the events in their life derive primarily from their own actions, while individuals with an external locus of control tend to blame others or their circumstances for their outcomes.

With this understanding, it's essential we develop a strong internal locus of control by accepting full responsibility for all our actions and inactions and resolving to do our best with what we have been given. By living from an internal locus of control, we will be a much more positive, upbeat and productive, and achieve more in our lives.

So, if you ever notice yourself feeling negative, helpless or stuck, resolve to get a firm hold of the situation and accepting full responsibility for creating the best outcome.

"If you don't design your own life plan, chances are you'll fall into someone else's plan. And guess what they have planned for you? Not much."
– Jim Rohn

2. Morning Power Hour – Reading

Get up one hour earlier in the morning and read an inspirational or motivational self-help book to put you into a high energy, positive frame of mind for the rest of your day. Another topic you could choose to read would be about your current industry or field of work. Over time, your knowledge, value and productivity will increase in your chosen occupation and you will be able to move up to higher levels in your profession.

You could also read other positive self-help books in other important life subjects to improve your personal abilities and skills. These other subjects for your to consider would be; relationships, communication, leadership, health, exercise, business, financial and personal development. A great book that I recommend for those of you interested in developing a powerful positive outlook that will serve you well throughout your life in both good and bad times is: *Success Through A Positive Mental Attitude* by W. Clement Stone.

This book has had a permanent lasting impact on how I think and live my life and will be very valuable to anyone who wants to become a more positive, strong upbeat individual. You really can choose how to respond to anything in life, *it's a choice*.

"Every day do something that will inch you closer to a better tomorrow."
– Doug Firebaugh

3. Morning Power Hour – Audio

When you wake up in the morning, kick-start your day powerfully by feeding your mind a breakfast of powerful motivational, inspirational or educational audio material. This can come in the form of audiobooks and mp3 tracks downloaded to your mp3 headset; you could listen to audio CDS while you drive to and from work in your car, or you could watch a motivational or inspirational video online.

All of these methods of feeding yourself with powerful input each morning during the first hour of your day will put you into a positive frame of mind and cause you to perform at your best throughout your day. Some excellent motivational and inspirational speakers that I recommend that you look into and listen to during your first waking hour of your day include: Brain Tracy, John C, Maxwell, Les Brown, Jim Rohn, Eric Thomas, Dr Wayne Dyer and Napoleon Hill. There are many more for you to look into and find out for yourself. Some speakers and teachers will relate with and add value to you more than others, the key is to find ones that give you a powerful charge of positive energy and incorporate them into your morning routine.

"You will never change your life until you change something you do daily."
   – Mike Murdock

3. Powerful Inner Circle

It is well known that as *humans, we become like those people we spend most of our time with.* Human beings tend to unconsciously become more and more like the people we associate with. People can influence our thinking, actions, habits and even beliefs. Therefore it's vital to surround ourselves with positive, success-oriented, like-minded people.

"Ask for help, not because you're weak, but because you want to remain strong."
   – Les Brown

5. Create a Growth Environment

We are all products of our environment although the great majority of us are completely unaware of how much our behaviours and thinking are influenced by those we choose to spend time with. Take a look around you. How are you spending your time? What environments are you putting yourself in? Are your co-workers negative, lazy and uninterested in their job?

Are the coaches at your sports club keen or do they seem like they don't want to be there? You could decide to look around your area, do your research and find out if there are any winning clubs or teams who are passionate and focused on producing results and winning. Take the time to speak with the club owners about your current situation and see if they would be able to help you.

If the situation is *win/win,* meaning that both you and the other club will gain value and benefit from this mutual association, then this may be the right choice for you. In your home, create a safe haven for you and your family. Your home should be a place where you can all relax, be yourself and rest from the outside work and everything that's going on in your lives.

Create a positive, open, supportive atmosphere towards your children and other family members. Never allow your home to be a limiting, criticising, abusive negative place. Make sure that your home is a positive growth environment that can build your family up, rather than tear each other down. In order to keep developing as a person, you must make sure that throughout your twenty-four hour days, each and every day, over the weeks and months and years ahead in your life, that you are constantly being positively inspired and influenced.

It's your role, and responsibility, to create an environment where the positive stimuli outweigh the negative. By getting and staying in this positive aura most of the time, you have put yourself into an environment conducive to achieving your goals and desires. You have created a growth environment.

"You are a product of your environment. So choose the environment that will best develop you toward your objective. Analyse your life in terms of its environment. Are the things around you helping you toward success – or are they holding you back?"
        – W. Clement Stone

6. Give Yourself Insanity Checks

Insanity is defined as: *"Doing the same thing, over and over again, yet expecting a different result."* Are you insane? Take a step outside of yourself for a moment as if you were watching yourself from across the street. Have you been unconsciously repeating the same actions day in and day out and then become discouraged or confused as to why you're not getting those results that you truly want for yourself when it comes to losing weight and shedding excess body fat?

If you've been repeating the same actions in your life, whether consciously or unconsciously, and you've not been getting the results you desire, then it's now time for a change. In order for you to achieve different results, you must *do something different or better.* You have to be open and be completely honest with yourself about your behaviour to change it. Starting from now, you can change the way you do things.

This may require a huge shift in your thinking and weekly routine, or it may even just take one simple idea or insight that you may have not yet been aware of. That's why it's vital to pay attention to the chapters in this book and intentionally seek information that could open a new door in your thinking. Once you discover a new, better way of doing things you will need to repeat these new behaviours to bring about consistent change.

"Insanity: doing the same thing over and over again and expecting different results."
        – Albert Einstein

1. Fail Forward

Failure is great. It shows that you're alive and you're trying. Learn from every little failure and setback along the path as you work towards your goal, adjusting your actions along the way. Many of us perceive failure as a negative thing, but failure is a tool and a signal to re-evaluate. We fail at most things before we get them right.

Analyse all your failures to take the valuable lesson from each one, and then try again in a slightly different way. Eventually you will have success. Les Brown, a famous motivational speaker (one of the best) states that: *anything worth doing in life is worth doing badly, until you learn how to do it well.* When you know what you want and have set the goal and made a full personal commitment to get it, you must be willing to do whatever it takes to achieve it.

All the failures along the way are there to *serve and teach you* how to succeed. If you find that the fear of failure is holding you back from trying new things and becoming successful in your life, I recommend that you buy John C. Maxwell's book: *Failing Forward.* The lessons and information in this book will change how you view failure and approach challenges forever. Your life will never be the same again.

> *"I've missed more than 9000 shots in my career. I've lost almost 300 games. 26 times, I've been trusted to take the game winning shot and missed. I've failed over and over and over again in my life. And that is why I succeed."*
> **– Michael Jordan**

Long Term Thinking – Embrace the Process of Change

It's very important to *think long term.* Think twenty years from now, how healthy would you like to be? What actions can you take now? While habits are not easy to change, it doesn't mean they're impossible to change. Throughout this book I will teach you many new habits, rituals, strategies, methods of exercising and nutritional principles to maximise your physique and energy levels.

For each of them there is a specific *process of learning* that you must fully embrace in order to implement and then convert them into new positive supportive habits in your life. This process of learning new skills and behaviours that will improve the overall quality of your life consists of four stages:

Stage 1: Unconscious Unknowing

This stage is when *you don't know that you don't know something.* For example, before you read it in a book, before you hear of it in a conversation, before your coach tells you about it. *You simply do not even know* that the new way of doing something even exists.

Stage 2: Conscious Unknowing

This stage is when you *now know that you don't know* about a certain subject or issue. This is when you decide you want to learn to improve your skills or ability. You know that there must be a better way of doing things; so you set out to find it – through books, people, schools, colleges, coaches, mentors etc.

Stage 3: Conscious Knowing

This is the stage when *you're now aware of a new improved way of doing something.* Although you've found it, you have *only just become aware of it and must now begin to put it into action* to bring about change.

Stage 4: Unconscious Knowing

This is the final stage of learning any new skill or improving any area or part of your life. *You have found out the solution to your problem and now understand how to do something better or in a way that will bring you the result that you want.* You have now been putting this solution into action in your life over and over again; practising until it starts to feel natural to you and you no longer need to invest so much of your energy into making it work. It begins to run on autopilot in your life and you can do it without even thinking about it.

You have *now created a new habit* and it will bring you the results and outcomes that you wanted. The key to mastering this fourth and final stage is *continuous action on a daily basis.* You need to keep repeating the new behaviour every day, week after week, until it finally locks in to your nervous system and becomes a very part of your being.

A perfect example of this process would be when you were learning to drive a car. At first you have to consciously think about everything: the clutch, the gear shift, the accelerator, and the visual checks. It's almost overwhelming and you will make mistakes and become frustrated. However by not giving up, continuing to invest your effort, attention, time and your energy into the process, one day soon you can drive without even thinking about it.

You can even have a conversation with somebody else sitting by your side and listen to the radio as you drive. This is the process of learning that I want you to acknowledge and apply to your efforts in changing your habits that contribute towards your physique and health. Realise that you will find it very difficult at the beginning. However it's your job to keep working at it, refer back to this book many times if you need to and just *keep on keeping on* until you eventually master each habit and skill.

Consider another time when you learned to play a musical instrument. Or learned to spell words and count numbers at school while you were a child. Think about the time you grew up, earning your degree and advancing through your profession with work experience and various jobs. Learning anything in life will follow this similar process.

It does not matter where you're currently at, or have been in your past, *all that matters is where you're going today and into your future.* The action that you are taking every single day: is it moving you closer to your goals and where you want to end up in life? Or is it moving you further away? You're the one in charge of your own results and your life.

You dont know how to do something.

You become aware that you dont know something.

You start to learn and practice what you know about. Yet progress is often slow, difficult and even frustating.

You kept repeating the action or behaviour consistently and did not give up. You have now found out what works and how to do it as a result of your own experience and it now becomes easy and natural for you. You have created a new habit. You can do it without even thinking/conscious attention.

Figure 4: The Process of Learning

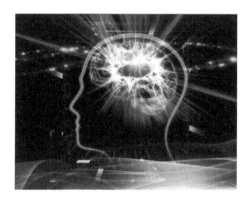

"The only source of knowledge is experience."
– Albert Einstein

Ride the Power of the Law of Attraction using your Brain

I have included a brief demonstration of the powerful universal Law of Attraction and how you can put it into action and get it to work in your life. The Law of Attraction is a well-known universal law that is always working in our lives whether we are conscious of it or not.

This law states that *everything we have in our lives at this or any moment and time we have attracted and drawn to us like a magnet by the predominant thoughts, feelings and our deepest desires that we hold in our minds and heart.*

When we understand the Law of Attraction, we can then use it as a *tool* to attract into our lives the things we *desire.* To activate this law, we must first know exactly, clearly, specifically *what we want in our lives.* We must then *truly believe that it's possible* for us to achieve it. Now with the goal set, and the belief that we *deserve,* and can *have it,* we activate the Law of Attraction to begin to work positively on our behalf.

The law will work closely with a particular organ located at the base of our brain called the Reticular Activating System or RAS. Our RAS's function is to alert us to everything in our environment and trigger ideas that can be used to move us closer to the attainment of a goal. Once we have been given the internal nudge, our gut feeling or intuition that a specific action must be taken in our lives; such as buying a particular book, attending a specific event, reaching out to a certain person, or signing up for a specific education course; the final step required is to activate the Law of Attraction.

By doing so we can *manifest* what we want. This is done through taking *action.* **Action** is the essential requirement to make everything work. However, acting once on a gut feeling is *not enough.* We must adopt the habit of repeatedly taking *continuous action,* hundreds and sometimes even thousands of times, day after day, until we finally achieve our desire. There is no telling how long we need to continue taking massive, consistent daily action in the direction of our desire until we ultimately achieve it.

Each goal, dream and circumstance is totally different for all of us, depending on the nature of the goal and the circumstance we currently find ourselves in. However we must have complete, unwavering faith, and keep on using the Law of Attraction, (the RAS in our brain) and *acting on every cue that we are given along the way that will move us closer to the attainment of our goal.*

Each baby step is important as they all build upon each other and move us onwards and upwards towards our final destination.

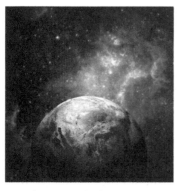

This may sound too complex for you to take in all at once and it often takes weeks or months of study to fully grasp and understand this process of manifesting desires in your life. However I will break the steps down for you to try and make the process easier to understand. That way you can begin putting this knowledge into action in your everyday life to bring you closer and closer to your goal – until you ultimately achieve it.

Step 1: Create within you a mental equivalent

Know exactly what it is that you want. Be 100% sure of what it is that you desire to *have, be, or achieve.* You have got to be very *specific.* This law will not work for anything if it's fuzzy or unclear in your mind. You must be definite about the thing or goal that you desire. Also, you must make sure that this is truly what you want from deep within your being and not what somebody else wants for you. It must be your own true inner desire.

When you know exactly what this is, create a vivid picture of you as if you have already attained it. This is known as *the mental equivalent.* The clearer and more vivid you can make this picture, the more power and energy you will have in your ability to manifest it in your life.

Step 2: Feel as if it's yours already, become the person capable of having it now. Hold the mental equivalent of exactly what you want in your mind as *if you already have it. Imagine the feeling of having it now* and how you would behave *every day* if you were that person. This raises your energy level, or *personal vibration* to match what you desire, strengthening your inner magnet and making you more receptive to all the people, events, materials, information and ideas around you which can move you closer to achieving it.

Step 3: Continually apply the Law of Action

Take *continual ongoing action;* every day that will move you closer and closer to achieving the mental equivalent you're holding in your mind. Take baby-steps, anything that will open new doors and paths in the direction of the thing you want. Know that what you want *also wants you* and that it's *simply a matter of taking all the actions day by day, step by step in the right direction.*

For example, to lose weight and look excellent, you must be taking action daily on things such as buying healthy nutritious foods at the shops, joining your local gym, putting in a workout session every day and so on. The steps don't need to be big, just little actions that will definitely move you in *the direction* of your end goal. Do not worry about this end goal or result just now, focus on taking constant, continuous actions *towards it.*

Think and act today as if you are already the person you are to become. What would you be doing if you were already that person?

Step 4: Focus on the Goal and not the Task

Keeping your focus on the end result as if you have already achieved it is known as *focusing on the goal.* Be flexible and open as you allow the universe to provide you with the quickest, easiest and shortest path to achieve your desire. Be open and receptive to the world around you and use what comes to you to bring you closer to your destination.

The way to attain what you want is different for everyone, your job is to allow that way to present itself to you and *act on it* as it appears. Draw from all the information, circumstances, people and ideas that come into your mind and current reality; things that can positively help and contribute towards you achieving your goal. Never let the vision of exactly what you want leave your mind.

Take these daily action steps and feel like the person you will be once you have achieved it. Keep your focus on taking the next step that opens up in front of you, no matter how big or small it may be. Listen to your intuition and the signals your Reticular Activating System at the base of your brain triggers within you. Act on the steps that feel right in moving you closer to your end goal with total faith.

Always remember, the key is that you don't have to see the whole picture of how it will all work out, all that you need to see or create is **the next step.** If you keep taking these next steps, then sooner or later the path will open up in front of you and you will arrive at your destination.

Step 5: Practice Intelligent Persistence

Stay in motion. Keep taking continual action on all *inspired ideas* that flash into your mind that will move you in the right direction. Act on all the information, resources and people around you that will bring you closer to what you want. Enjoy yourself along the way. Just continue to eat better, read more on the subject of exercise and nutrition, make friends with positive like-minded people, attend classes, and hire that personal trainer.

Do whatever is needed to help you to grow, improve, learn and become the person you need to be to achieve the end result. During this process, never waiver from your belief and conviction, that it's yours to be attained by demonstrating intelligent persistence. Intelligent persistence is the act of never giving up. However, as you begin making progress and mistakes along the way, *be aware of your mistakes, learn from them, and then try again more intelligently.*

Step 6: Become the person within, to create the reality without

By focusing on improving your current life situation and by holding that vision of yourself as if you have already achieved your goal, you *will* finally achieve it. And who knows, you may even surpass it by achieving more than you ever thought possible. The key to this process is to never stop believing in what you want and continuing to maximise your efforts towards what you want each and every day, always trying to do and be better today than you were yesterday. When you become that person, through your learning and experience, you will attract the situation and life that matches **who you are**. What they say is true, "you don't get in life what you want, you get in life *who you are*". You need to become the person capable of achieving what you desire and living the life you want to live, and then *it will come to you.*

Put your Reticular Activating System to work alongside the Law of Attraction to attract everything into your life that you desire.

> *"Take the first step in faith. You don't have to see the whole staircase, just take the first step."*
> **– Martin Luther King Jr**

Visualise and Positively Affirm Yourself Along The Way

Another excellent *tool* that you can use is the power of *visualisation.* Learn and develop your ability to visualise yourself as a lighter, leaner version of yourself, eating a complete nutritious diet, cleansing your body with plenty of water and walking around each day looking in superb physical condition. Whatever your goal, visualise yourself enjoying the rewards of its successful outcome.

Truly believe and feel as if you are in the process right now, of becoming this version of yourself. Make method visualisation a frequent habit in moments that you have to spare throughout your day. This will then create a positive charge of energy within you and align yourself with many of the powerful universal laws that will work in your favour.

You may begin to feel or see yourself as getting lucky as certain coincidences start appearing in your life that pull you closer and closer to attaining that which you desire. Perform these visualisations often enough, while keeping your focus on massive daily **action,** and before long you will manifest this vision in your physical reality.

Don't get discouraged when you don't get things right away. By staying consistent in your efforts, you will soon trick your mind into thinking that you are already that lean and trim person, and you will start to take actions each day that will make sure you become that person.

Wake up each morning, step on the scales, notice the weight has dropped and then picture yourself in the mirror as a much leaner, lighter and well defined version of yourself. Keep this positive visualisation and forward thinking habitual during specific moments of your day. What you can see clearly in your mind, you also have the power inside yourself to hold in your hand.

As for affirmations, they need to be true, your own, short, heartfelt, and emotionally charged from within your being. You need to *feel them* all over your body as you declare them to yourself, whether out loud, or in your internal self-talk. The key to making affirmations work for you is to use them only after experiencing a small victory or successful outcome that pushes you in the direction of your end goal or desire.

For example, during the time of my life when my main focus and desire was to become the best amateur boxer that I could be, and win as many bouts as possible, each night after a great training session, where I pushed myself to my limits and performed in excellent fashion, I would make an affirmation. I would say with *power and conviction* to myself that I was "unstoppable, ruthless, strong, ferocious, in great shape, the best…"

By continuing this practice, naturally each time you experience a small win, you begin to train your subconscious mind to create a new and improved belief system within yourself, causing all your actions on the outside to improve and be more in alignment with the goals and desires that you have set for yourself. Use and practice the habit of frequent visualisation and affirmations as *tools,* on your journey from where you are to where you want to be.

"Whatever the mind can conceive and believe, it can achieve."
– Napoleon Hill

The Zone

In your quest you will experience setbacks, mistakes and temporary failures. This is an *inevitable* part of the process. The most important thing for you to do during these times is to find a way to bring yourself back to 'the zone'. Never get caught up on your mistakes or past experiences. It's the past and you no longer live there.

How do you bring yourself back to the zone? Let's say for example, you have been eating great quality, nutritious meals in moderate portion sizes at the right times over the last two days. Today for whatever reason, you slip up and fall off the course of your good eating by drinking a sweetened coffee and slice of cake that was a treat from a friend.

Okay, you may have slipped up temporarily, however *you must bring yourself back to the zone* by waiting four hours and making sure that when you begin to feel hungry again that your next meal is a healthy, nutrient dense, low calorie meal. After eating a good meal that's more in alignment with your goal you put yourself back into the zone. You have created a clean slate and must now focus your attention on making more and more positive progress towards losing weight, losing body fat and getting as lean as you can again.

Acknowledge that you may have slipped out of the zone and, if you can, try to reduce the potential for it happening again. This could be thanking your relative and letting them know that you don't want them to bring you any more cake in the future and explain why. Once back in the zone, **stay there.**

What is important here is never to be overly hard on yourself, feel guilty, become negative or beat yourself up whenever you make the occasional slip up in your nutrition, exercise or any other area in your life. It is completely normal. Recognise that you have slipped up, remind yourself that you will be more conscious and aware in future situations and then put it behind you. You will soon have a great sense of control over yourself and your life again.

"The successful person has the habit of doing the things failures don't like to do. They don't like doing them either necessarily. But their disliking is subordinated to the strength of their purpose."
– E. M. Gray

Make Progress The Goal Of All of Your Goals

Setting goals for weight loss can lead to disappointment so I prefer to set goals in terms of exercise planning, but not defining how much weight will be lost or inches shed. I prefer to focus on progress. Progress should always be your goal. You will never be perfect; however you can always be better today than you were yesterday. **Progress** is measured on scales or body composition machines at a local health club.

You could even just use how you look and feel when you look in the mirror each morning. You will surely know that you're making progress if you begin to receive compliments from the people around you. Keep your attention focused on constant action and improvement in your nutrition and exercise efforts and routine. I find when we set goals related to our bodies, we tend to spend too much time checking, analysing and thinking about how we look, when all that time and energy should be focused on doing the things that will bring us the results.

Instead of checking on a sheet of paper all the time, and over analysing whether or not you're doing well, get to the gym, go for a jog, focus at your sports club or go on a bike trip with the family. Get busy living and enjoying your life so much that you don't have time to sit and analyse health and fitness goals. When you look in the mirror your results will speak for themselves.

I do believe in the power of goals; however leave them up to the personal trainers or other people. You want to use your daily exercise tracker presented earlier to measure your progress in terms of how much time you spend each week being active rather than stepping on the scales. Your **actions** are the only thing that will bring you the results you want. That's why I want you to pass on goals and focus all your precious time and *energy in action*. You see, getting into the best shape of your life should not be a goal. It should be a lifestyle, a way of life. You must keep your focus on learning and progress, so that you can live and breathe the habits and actions required for you. If you set goals, while you might reach them, you might also fall back into lazy patterns and habits which could cause you to end up back where you started. You need to learn to focus on *continual progress and improvement* and that way you will be able to maintain an excellent well defined physique on a permanent basis for the rest of your life.

> *"Success is the progressive realization of a worthy goal or ideal"*
> **– Earl Nightingale**

Become Aware of Them then Shoot Down Self-limiting Beliefs

Life creates self-limiting beliefs. These are the beliefs that hold us in the same place and prevent us from moving forward. When we were children, we were all great dreamers. We believed anything was possible if we truly wanted it. As we grew up things changed.

Our parents, teachers, school systems and negative influences around us in society began to unconsciously program us with doubts and untrue self-limiting beliefs about who we are and what were truly capable of. Recognise these moments in your past that may have shaped you, and realise that you may still be holding onto beliefs that are *untrue*. Just the act of recognising these moments and how they shaped you can bring about change.

To transcend your old self-imposed self-limiting beliefs, you must decide to take positive action in your present situation. Action is the key to change. Recognise that some limitations are self-imposed and therefore can be altered.

"Nothing can stop the man with the right mental attitude from achieving his goal; nothing on earth can help the man with the wrong mental attitude."
– Thomas Jefferson

Become Aware to Have the Power

In order to change or improve anything in your life you must first know that something you're doing is not helping you achieve your goals or even moving you further away from them. So the first stage is to *become aware.* This awareness is the first step to creating a new improved way of doing things.

Let's take for example that you are having problems and trouble losing weight. You are not making noticeable lasting progress. When you take a look back at your actions over the day you realise that you frequently binge during the evenings on a whole bar of chocolate after your evening meal.

By honestly questioning, and looking deep inside yourself to try and find out the true underlying cause for this behaviour, you may discover that this eating had nothing to do with physically being hungry. In fact you may realise that you were compelled to eat for an emotional reason. Whether you have been feeling lonely, sad, bored or had a stressful day at work, it is the ability to view yourself objectively that will allow you to see what to address for change.

Rather than turning to the kitchen cupboard trying to solve your emotional issues with chocolates, you will take constructive action towards *the real issue.* This may be discussing issues at work, visiting family or friends for a chat and some good company or putting on a funny DVD. The answer is never food. Food will only make things worse, causing you to feel guilty and even more negative and helpless towards yourself and your situation.

It's all about awareness. So if you're not looking lean with a low level of total body fat, maybe you're not eating the right kinds of foods. You may be eating too many carbohydrates and not enough proteins and vegetables during the second part of your day. The more you practise becoming aware of yourself: how you think, how you act and why you do what you do, the easier it will be to find solutions.

Apply Awareness in Your Life:

Step 1:

Take a look at yourself and your daily behaviours as if you were watching yourself from the outside. Become aware of the actions or behaviours that you may be engaging in throughout your day that will be counterproductive to achieving the best physique you're capable of. Grab a notebook or piece of paper and a pen and write the numbers 1 to 10 down the left hand side of the page. Beside each number write down the behaviour that you can think of that you engage in throughout your day that may be preventing you from getting great results in your weight loss, physique or health goals. Once you have spent five or ten minutes reflecting on your day or week and picked out those actions that you know have been holding you back, you will have made yourself more aware of your behaviours. Simply by this act of becoming more aware, you will now have *more control over the choice you make* when faced with these similar actions or problems in your future.

Step 2:

Work to replace the limiting behaviours that may be holding you back from looking and feeling your best with a more constructive opposite behaviour that will move you towards your goals and fire up your rate of progress faster than you can imagine. A few small changes, in the right areas can lead to dramatic changes in your results.

You can use this method of self-analysis over and over again throughout the progress of working towards your goals in your life. Simply remove or replace the behaviours and actions that you're consciously or unconsciously taking throughout your current routine and watch the positive effect it will have on your results and ability to achieve all your goals you have set for yourself.

The starting point of all positive change and improvement in your life is awareness. Become aware of why you are acting that way and doing the things you are doing. As humans, we are 95% creatures of habit. Most of our ways of acting are conditioned behaviours. Question yourself before you perform a behaviour or pattern of behaviour and then stop anything that is preventing you from achieving your goals. Replace them with more positive, new supportive behaviours instead.

You will soon learn to make these positive behavioural changes permanent or new habit patterns by rewiring your nervous system through repetition so that the negative patterns lose their strength, while your new improved behaviours will start to run on autopilot.

Why do you do what you do? Why do you eat overly big portions or choose second helpings? Why do you always eat cakes and biscuits when offered every time you visit a friend or relative? Why do you eat too much food during the evenings, destroying your chance to get into that essential negative energy balance that's required to lose weight? **The more awareness we have the more control we take.**

"There is nothing noble about being superior to some other man. The true nobility is in being superior to your previous self."
– Hindu Proverb

All Causation is Mental

It all begins and ends in the mind. Your body is simply a physical reflection of all the choices you have made over your lifetime up to the present moment. The two things that you have full control over are *what you eat* and *how much you exercise*. Figure 4 shows how your mind-set should be focused on these two factors as these will determine the results; i.e. in achieving the greatest physique you possibly can.

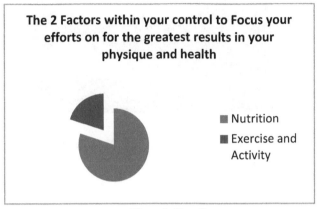

Figure 5: Your Focus

"Shoot for the moon and if you miss you will still be among the stars."
 – Les Brown

Continually Educate Yourself

As you take positive action from what you learn from this book, you will keep on learning. Use everything positive that you learn from reading or listening. This will further accelerate your progress. The more you know, the better the results. New ideas breed further learning and will prompt you to try out other new things. *Change is the only constant in life.* Science is evolving; we, as humans, are evolving. Ten years from today everything you see around you will have changed. There will be newer, more effective and productive ways to do things, so it's your job to *go with the changes.* Never stop learning.

"Reading is to the mind what exercise is to the body."
 – Joseph Addison

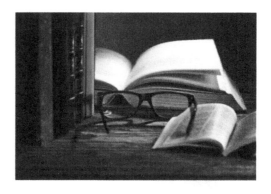

"Once your mind-set changes, everything on the outside will change along with it."
– Steve Maraboli

Summary:

• **Create within yourself a Mental Equivalent** of the ideal you would like to become in terms of your physical appearance and feeling of good health. Keep this vision in your mind as you begin to make positive changes and continue to take constructive action towards your goals that will affect how you will look and feel.

• **Activate the Law of Attraction and the Reticular Activating System** in your brain and then keep taking action on all the cues that show up in your path along the way in alignment with your goals towards your destination.

• **Identify, then shoot down any Self-Limiting Beliefs** you may have holding you back from making progress in losing weight and improving your level of health. Then once you have become aware, take positive constructive action to transcend these old, learned beliefs in order to gain new positive experiences to develop new, supportive beliefs that will produce greater results for you in your future.

- **Understand and then embrace the Process of Learning** that is required in learning new skills and behaviours and that will contribute towards the attainment of your goals.

- **Resolve to listen to five audio books or CDs** related to your goals that will give you new valuable information that could improve that area of your life when put into action. Consider your health, career, positive thinking, leadership, time-management or any other area that will positively influence your life.

- **Resolve to read five books related to your goals** that will give you new valuable information that could improve that area of your life when put into action. Consider your health, career, positive thinking, leadership, time-management or any other area that will positively influence your life.

-7-

Supplements

Why Supplement?

Many people have forgotten the true reason for taking dietary supplements. More and more health stores are opening on high streets selling hundreds, even thousands, of products we just don't need. Internet sites sell and distribute products, with *larger than life* claims, promising amazing results in: burning body fat, losing weight, building muscle and curing all our health problems.

If it sounds too good to be true: it probably is. Supplements should only be used *when needed* and *with guidance*. The dictionary defines a supplement as: *"something added to complete a thing, supply a deficiency, or reinforce/extend a whole"*. Take note of these three phases.

We can imagine completing something in the context of what we eat. If our meals are 'incomplete' or 'out of balance' they are missing an important component needed for optimal health and body composition. For example protein or omega-3 fatty acids and so then supplementation can be seen as *completing a thing.*

Supplying a deficiency similarly means a nutrient is missing, in this case routinely from the diet perhaps from dislike of a key food, inability or absorb a key ingredient or accidently omitted; perhaps the result of poor dietary choices. Deficiencies can lead to diseases and so supplements can be used/prescribed.

Using a supplement *to reinforce or extend a whole* illustrates their role in strengthening what is already present. An example would be the use of a small amount of caffeine to further stimulate mental capacity or physical activity ability. But choosing supplements requires guidance and what works for one might not work for someone else. That's why it's important to consider your own personal goals, circumstances and always seek medical/expert advice.

Despite cunning marketing and sales claims, no single supplement will produce instant results. Around 90% or more of the supplements marketed today will produce absolutely no visible, or health benefit whatsoever. Of these 90%, the great majority will actually do you harm. Only a very small number, 5–10% of the supplements marketed today actually appear to have any effect in serving their purpose and promoting the activity they claim on their labels. Take care with those fat burning or *magic pills* you see advertised.

Most of your foods will give you what you need and supplements are for specific cases where something is missing, not absorbed or is known to have a positive benefit. Otherwise, clean healthy eating; regular consistent physical activity and a positive state of mind will work better than many of these pills!

If you're suffering from a particular health problem then seek the advice of a doctor and be aware of your diet, don't take something based on the manufacturer's claims as you may do more harm. Do your research and find out if you need something before you even consider taking it. It is important that you understand when, why and how to use dietary supplements.

Use this chapter as a reference, a guide to a few of the recognised and traditionally used supplements known to enhance your body composition, health status and physical and mental performance.

Protein Powder Supplements

Whey protein powders, casein protein powders and vegetable protein powders are all simply powdered forms of food which we can eat in order to gain protein for growth and repair of muscles, cells and other functions within our body. They may be powdered forms of the food we eat, but they are not always as good as the food we eat.

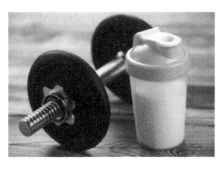

Fresh, whole food sources of protein always provide us with more value per gram in terms of nutrition as they are free from flavourings, sugars and other processing chemicals often added to these powdered forms. Yet there are times where we can all benefit from including protein powder into our meals at some time during our day. For example, to maximise weight loss, body fat reduction, lean muscle growth, lean muscle maintenance and high physical strength and vitality levels.

A fresh fruit salad is an excellent choice of meal for weight loss to have for our breakfast, yet without a lean source of protein we would be putting our bodies at risk if we've not consumed protein in the past eight hours since sleeping. We could add protein by topping the fruit with a couple of spoons of low-fat natural yoghurt or a flavoured whey protein mixture.

You could similarly *complete* a bowl of porridge or low-sugar breakfast cereal the same way. A meal of carbohydrates alone without adequate amounts of protein to balance it out on a regular, ongoing basis is the surest way to shift your body into a fat storage machine. This is why whey protein is the most popular dietary supplement.

Whey & Casein Protein

There are two main different types of protein; here we will discuss: **whey** and **casein**. Whey protein is absorbed into our bodies and transported to our muscles at a much quicker rate than casein which tends to get transported and used within our bodies over a longer period of time. This is why all bodybuilders and high level athletes tend to consume a whey protein shake after their workouts in order to speed up the recovery process.

Casein protein however, is much harder to break down and tends to supply our muscles gradually over a period of a few hours.

This can be useful if one is experiencing a high level of physical hunger later at night, especially before bed time. By consuming a casein powder mixed with some water in a shake, you would continue to feed your muscles and burn off excess body fat while you sleep.

Vegan and Vegetarian Protein Powders

Any vegetarians looking to incorporate more lean protein into their daily meals should also consider using protein supplements. There are a variety of different protein powders they can choose from such as soy, hemp, brown rice, pea egg and some other forms. If considering including any vegetable or dairy based protein powders, consider doing your research first in order to make sure you get yours from a high quality source from a reputable brand best suited to your goals and requirements.

Protein Shakes & Bars

It should never be your intention to drink a protein shake instead of a meal. Whole food, nutritious balanced meals should always be the key focus. However, there will be times when having a meal every four hours isn't possible and so you turn to this as an alternative. The key to getting the most benefit from your protein is to combine your protein powder with water, rather than its higher calorie alternative: milk. If you happen to be a highly active individual with a larger body frame, then you may require more calories than the average man or women, therefore milk can be used. However, a whey protein and water shake is one of the best snack options possible as it fully promotes a lean physique by feeding your muscles and keeping the metabolism in good working order thus promoting the fat burning ability of your body.

Quality First

When selecting your protein powder, to implement into your current routine, whether combining with your meals, as a snack, or as an *on the go* shake during busy times, the important thing for you to look out for is *quality*. The quality of your protein is the most important factor to consider. Always buy popular, well known brands that provide high quality lean protein.

Non-denatured whey protein is the higher quality type you should be looking for if possible as the protein powder will be much higher in bio locally active peptides. Do your research; don't always shop for the lowest price protein you can find. Read the labels and look for key ingredients and ensure that you get a high return of protein per gram.

A great blend that I personally use is *P.H.D diet whey protein* as it contains many natural healthy ingredients and compounds such as green tea catechins, ground flaxseeds, CLA and L-Carnitine which all work to promote health, fat burning and weight loss.

Omega-3 Fatty Acids for Fat Burning

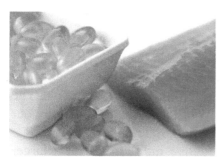

We have already discussed the use of omega-3 in our diets and the importance of supplementation to maintain the correct omega-3:6 ratio. Another benefit is its direct role in promoting fat burning. Omega-3 promotes the activity of fat burning genes and in minimising the storage of fat in our bodies. It does this by increasing our insulin sensitivity.

Glucosamine Sulphate, Chondroitin and MSM

As we age the cartilage that cushions our joints to allow pain free, fluid, flexible movement begins to wear. Highly active athletes can also suffer this due to unnatural stresses on joints and signs include: joint stiffness, pains or even movement limitations in specific areas like our ankles, knees, hips, wrists, elbows and shoulders.

This will limit every day movements like bending down, lifting objects, even walking. However thanks to the natural supplements like glucosamine sulphate, chondroitin and MSM we can control this to some extent.

Glucosamine Sulphate

Glucosamine helps to renew, protect, revitalise, rejuvenate and nourish cartilage. Glucosamine is a key element of cartilage itself and provides building blocks to construct new cartilage. Our body naturally produces very small amounts of glucosamine but since this diminishes with age the need for supplementation increases.

Chondroitin

Chondroitin, like glucosamine, is also a key structural component of cartilage and when used as a supplement helps in renewing, revitalising, rejuvenating and maintaining joints. Chondroitin also promotes synovial fluid secretion into joints which assists joint mobility.

Methylsulfonylmethane (MSM)

MSM is an organic source of sulphur which is a mineral that is vital in the formation of collagen, connective tissue and healthy cartilage around our joints. Sulphur is a powerful ingredient that nourishes our joints and protects against joint discomfort.

If you experience joint issues, especially as you age, seek medical advice as there are a number of other supplements available to you that might help. For example, collagen and hyaluronic acid. Collagen is a glue-like substance that helps form cartilage by holding all the cartilage building blocks together and giving the cartilage its shock-absorbing capabilities that reduce wear and tear.

Collagen is a critical structural element of healthy cartilage and research has proven that collagen, when taken consistently, and combined with healthy joint promoting habits and nutrition, helps to reduce pain experienced from osteoarthritis as well as supporting the health of our cartilage.

Hyaluronic acid is also another effective supplement that will help to cushion our joints by promoting the production of joint lubricating synovial fluid. This reduces the overall effects of wear and tear.

There are also powerful supplement *blends* available that combine all three of the most effective joint health promoting ingredients: glucosamine, chondroitin and MSM. Some also include collagen, hyaluronic acid and other similar agents. These are available in liquid or tablet form and can be taken with any of your meals. Seek advice as you might really benefit from finding the right one if you have issues with your joints.

Long Term Joint Heath

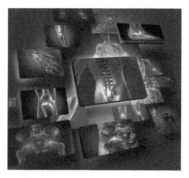
There is no doubt that a *combination* of healthy diet, light to moderate exercise and the guided use of supplements can help you to maintain healthy joints as you age. Joint health is promoted by foods rich in antioxidants like omega-3 fish oil, fresh vegetables, fruits and green tea and spices with anti-inflammatory properties, such as ginger and turmeric.

Light physical activities such as walking, swimming and cycling are great for joints. The key is to *stay in motion* and keep those joints working to maximise mobility, flexibility and keep them strengthened. A body in motion tends to stay in motion, while a body at rest tends to stay at rest.

Reduction of some foods from the diet will also help; for example inflammatory food and drinks containing sugar, alcohol or caffeine such as sweets, cakes, syrups, fizzy drinks, alcoholic beverages as well as strong coffees and processed junk foods.

Follow these guidelines and you will create a powerful synergistic effect and promote healthy joints.

Multivitamins/Multiminerals

For those who live very active lifestyles, consume insufficient volumes of fresh vegetables or fruit, consume too many processed/junk foods or are immunocompromised, supplementing with multivitamins and minerals may be a good idea. The nutrient levels will not be as good quality as from the food itself and changing bad habits is the best way to good health. However these are available and may help in some situations.

Multivitamins and minerals are usually taken before meals; one or two daily but always follow the manufacturer's recommended daily dosage or you may experience nausea, diarrhoea, stomach cramps and a range of other issues related to the toxic effects of excess. As well as these side effects, exceeding dosage carries no benefit as the body can only effectively absorb a certain volume or the vitamin/mineral and will be excreted if in excess.

Greens

A greens supplement might be needed if your diet does not contain sufficient vegetables and fruits. This can lead to a hormonal imbalance that is not only destructive to weight loss but is not good for optimal health. Whether you're on a busy work or travel schedule, or are simply one of those fussy people who refuse to eat a variety of healthy nutritious vegetables and fruits, then greens supplements could be for you.

But be aware that changing to better eating habits is always the preferable way. If you feel you would benefit from a few scoops of greens powder each day then do your research and then purchase a quality product.

Implementation

Have a look at the action plan outlined below. Only use supplements if you really need them!

Action Plan:

Chosen Supplement	How it can benefit my health, weight loss, fat loss, muscle building or performance level	When to consume in my daily routine	Implemented into my routine to accelerate my progress towards my goals. ☑
			☐
			☐
			☐
			☐

-8-

Positive Life Habits

"Your beliefs become your thoughts,
Your thoughts become your words,
Your words become your actions,
Your actions become your habits,
Your habits become your values,
Your values become your destiny."
– Mahatma Gandhi

Our Habits either Make or Break us

Habits shape our behaviour from a very young age, some good, some destructive, some just because we have always acted that way. But as humans we have the ability to become *conscious* of how we think and therefore how we choose to act. This means that all habits are transitory, we can change them.

We brush our teeth every day, we drive or take the bus to work each day, we eat roughly the same foods, engage in the same activities and passions, spend time around the same set of people and so on. Recognising habits, especially those that are not beneficial, even harmful, means we can learn to replace them.

We do this by reprogramming our actions for a minimum of twenty-one days, day after day until we have created a new habit. To succeed on a permanent basis, it is simply a matter of reprogramming. We need to begin consciously by shifting our mind-set until it becomes automatic.

"We become what we repeatedly do."
– Sean Covey

Positive Life Habits to Implement:

Go Heavy on the Green Tea

Drinking around *3 – 5* cups of Green Tea over the period of your day will slightly increase your body's ability to burn body fat while being physically active and at rest. The thermic effect from drinking green has a great impact on raising our metabolism and by drinking between *3 – 5* cups, every few hours over the course of our day, we burn around 50 – 100 calories alone simply from the effects of our increased metabolism. A type of catechin prevalent in green tea, epigallocatechin gallate (EGCG), raises our resting metabolism and stimulates fat-burning *within* the cells of our bodies. A small positive change like this will greatly contribute towards your weight loss.

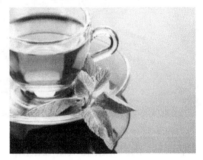

Morning Power Hour

Supercharge your day by giving your mind a powerful mental warm up during the vital first hour of your day. The first hour of your day is when your brain is fresh and most vulnerable to whatever stimuli it's exposed to. Feed your mind by reading a good book or listening to positive mp3 audio tracks of motivational, inspirational or educational material as you awaken, you set yourself up for your day.

By combining listening to powerful audio material with your daily tasks or activities during this first hour such as a morning walk or jog, housework, meal preparation, you will put yourself in a positive frame of mind, making you more focused, productive and positive throughout the rest of the day.

"As you begin changing your thinking, start immediately to change your behavior. Begin to act the part of the person you would like to become. Take action on your behavior. Too many people want to feel, then take action. This never works."
— **John Maxwell**

Clean Eating Lifestyle

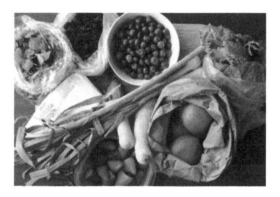

Develop the habit of eating only clean, fresh, whole, natural nutritious foods. Live on a very nutrient dense, low calorie diet. Create within yourself a strong dislike of greasy, fattening fast foods and increase your experience of cooking and eating your own delicious, tasty nutritious meals. Only load fresh, whole, single-ingredient foods into your shopping basket while at the supermarket.

Visit local fishmongers, butchers and farm shops to buy fresh, lean quality protein foods and fresh fruit and vegetables that are loaded with essential nutrients. *Make your home your greatest asset* by only ever bringing into it fresh, highly nutritious food and rejecting anything that will sabotage your efforts of being the leanest, healthiest person that you can be.

Garnish your home with an exotic bowl of fruits to serve as an excellent decoration, while ensuring that when tempted, you snack on the good stuff rather than any processed junk. Make every effort you can that will create a positive environment of clean, healthy foods around you in your home. Remember the rule; *you cannot eat what's not within your reach.*

> *"Man Is What He Eats."*
> **– Lucretius**

Avoid the Three White Poisons

Eliminate **salt, sugar,** and **white flour products** as discussed in (Chapter 3: Nutrition)

> *"Garbage in garbage out."*
> **– George Fuechsel**

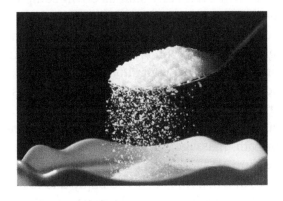

Remove all Processed Foods from your Diet

Any food that comes in a packet, wrapper or tin should be removed from the diet. These foods have all been processed to increase shelf life which means many of the essential nutrients have been removed and replaced with toxins and other substances that are not good for us. In the long term the accumulation of these products can produce health problems and reduce the length of our lives. So eliminate processed foods and eat only real food.

"Processed foods not only extend the shelf life, but they extend the waistline as well."
– Karen Sessions

Routinely Relax and De-stress

Being stressed causes our body to produce more of the stress hormone cortisol which increases our appetite and can lead to emotional eating or binging. If our current routines are inducing stress, our health will be jeopardised in both the long and short term. Stress is one of the biggest killers. Studies have shown that the majority of people suffer their first major heart attack between 8 and 9am on Monday morning.

Many of us are unhappy in our jobs. Being unhappy, anxious, worried or fearful will eventually shut us down completely. Take the time to become aware of the major causes of stress in your life, and the ways you can recognise your responses to it and therefore act to change. Recognise the price you are paying for not taking deliberate action in seeking a solution to your situation.

Some methods you could use in order to de-stress in your daily and weekly routine could include; going for a walk, vigorous exercise, yoga, stretching, meditation, listening to peaceful music, having a warm bath, massage, watch a funny film or comedy, do the gardening, take time off work, go on a vacation, and spend more time doing the hobbies and activities that you enjoy and love to do.

What I believe to be the single most effective technique in dealing with stress and removing it from any particular area of your life is to write the problem down on a piece of paper, seek to understand it and then create an action plan to reduce or eliminate it. These action steps could be asking for a different job role, more on-the-job training, a different level of responsibility at your work, changing how you spend your time in your social life, incorporating more relaxation and time for yourself to bring yourself back to your own grounded centre, a new career path or simply decluttering your life. Make it your own personal resolution to put your own inner peace before any other factor.

"Health is like money, we never have a true idea of its value until we lose it."
– Josh Billings

Move. Get Active.

"Physical fitness is not only one of the most important keys to a healthy body; it is the basis of dynamic and creative intellectual activity."
– John F. Kennedy

Learn and Develop your own Healthy Eating Cooking Skills.

Eating is one *constant* in all of our lives, so learning how to become an effective cook with a wide inventory of delicious meals will have lifelong benefits. Resolve to cook a new meal every week for yourself, spouse, family or friends. With every new meal you cook your experience in preparing, cooking and fine dining will be improving at a rapid pace.

"To eat is a necessity, but to eat intelligently is an art."
– La Rochefoucauld

Get Enough Sleep.

It is essential that we all get a good night of quality sleep to feel and function optimally. Sleep is essential for our body, mind and spirit to heal, repair and regenerate. Sleep is also the main requirement in growth and repair of your muscles, cells and systems of your body. Your goal should be to ensure you get a minimum of six hours of quality sleep every day, eight hours being a good target for most of us.

However as we are all different, some of us may be able to function at optimal levels on less sleep, while others may require a little more. The important thing is to have an awareness of our own needs. If our schedules, goals and responsibilities prevent us from getting a full night of good quality, undisturbed sleep, then I recommend a nap during the day. Afternoon siestas prove to be very effective in promoting many health benefits.

> *"The first wealth is health."*
> **– Ralph Waldo Emerson**

Be Religious about the Night Time Caloric Deficit

Stop eating after your evening meal, ideally from 5–6pm. Once your evening meal is finished, the kitchen is now closed, no excuses. The only exception would be a high quality lean protein snack later on during the evening only if you find yourself in a state of strong physical hunger.

Make this a habit as natural as breathing in and out by making it your new way of thinking and living each day; and you will have mastered one of the main techniques of being slim and trim for the rest of your life.

> *"What you eat in private will show up in public."*
> **– Unknown**

Constantly Feed Your Mind with the Right Stuff

If you read at least one motivational or educational book a month, that's twelve or more books a year. If you can read one book a week, that's fifty-two books a year which means the rate of growth you will experience in both your personal and professional life as well as in your overall development will be exceptional.

Why not build your own personal library of all the books that you have enjoyed reading that positively changed your way of thinking and how you live your life. Every one of us should build and forge out our own powerful philosophy of life through our own experiences and reflection. Reading books, listening to audio CDs, mp3 tracks, attending seminars and continually feeding our minds with powerful information, then applying what you learn is the key to improving your life experience.

"If you wish to achieve worthwhile things in your personal and career life, you must become a worthwhile person in your own self-development."
– Brian Tracy

Enrol in Never-ending Self-education

In order to improve any area of your life, you must first improve your knowledge and level of consciousness in that particular area so that you can act in more productive, higher quality ways in your everyday life. Read, study, understand, apply, and then make it a habit. Even the smallest, slightest improvements and changes in your routine will carry long-term benefits. Find what works for you and keep doing it.

Personal development is the secret to your success in life. Don't believe everything you hear, read or learn, not even from the so called experts until you have *given it a try* for yourself and discovered whether or not it's right for you and your situation. Develop your own tried and tested system through your own practical experiences over the course of your lifetime through continual learning, implementation and reflection.

"Give a man a fish and you feed him for a day. Teach a man to fish and you feed him for a lifetime."
– Chinese Proverb

Surround Yourself with Winners

As humans, we tend to unconsciously adopt all the behaviours, actions and attitudes of the people we spend the majority of our time with. As the old saying goes "Birds of the feather flock together." To take full advantage of this fact of human nature, you want to ensure that you surround yourself with positive, upbeat people who build you up rather than tear you down. Supportive, non-judgemental people who love and accept you unconditionally for who you are and what you stand for in your life. Surround yourself with the best and with time you will soon become one of the best yourself.

> *"There are two primary choices in life: to accept conditions as they exist, or accept the responsibility for changing them."*
> **– Dr. Denis Waitley**

Be Organised

Plan your meals a week in advance, not down to the exact calorie but taking into consideration the quality of nutrients. You want to gain the maximum amount of nutrition in relation to the number of calories you consume. Plan to purchase and eat only nutrient dense, fresh, whole, organic meats, poultry, fish, fruits, vegetables and whole-grains.

Plan your exercise and physical activities for the month ahead on your exercise calendar. Plan your working responsibilities and duties for the day in advance. Plan your yearly time off from work and family vacations in advance. Plan everything that is important to you, your goals and the main people in your life in advance. The more organised you are, the more control you will have over your life, your time and the results you produce.

This will make you a more positive, productive, less stressed, happier person who gets more out of your time spent here in this one shot at life you've been gifted with.

> *"Motivation is what gets you started. Habit is what keeps you going."*
> **– Jim Rohn**

Strive to Live a Balanced Life

Our life consists of many different areas that are important to our wellbeing, optimal functioning and quality of life. Being out of balance in just one of these areas can cause us to become stressed, unhappy and unfulfilled.

Areas such as work, play, family, relationships, financial status, rest, recreation, health and spirituality all have a major role in our lives and when we find any one of them is in danger or out of balance it negatively affects us in many ways.

That's why it's essential that you manage to engage in activities that positively contribute to each important area of your life and discipline yourself to refrain from negative behaviours. The more balanced your life is in each area, the more content you will feel.

"First we make our habits and then our habits make us."
– John Dryden

Negative Lifestyle Habits to Avoid:

Getting into a Mess

It's simple: if you are in a state of positive energy balance at the end of each day you will gain weight and accumulate excess body fat. This particularly applies to the second part of your day, where it's essential that you cut down on the amount of foods you eat after your evening meal.

Many factors contribute to 'getting into this mess': emotions, stress levels, influences, environment, self-discipline and so on. Awareness of your own bad habits is the first step towards change.

"The only way to keep your health is to eat what you don't want, drink what you don't like, and do what you'd rather not."
– Mark Twain

Junk Food

Get all of the Trans fats, packaged foods, microwave foods, ready-made meals, hydrogenated vegetable oils, high saturated fatty foods, fast food takeaways, crisps, sweats, cakes, soft drinks out of your diet. Don't eat them. It's that simple.

> *"Don't eat anything your great-great grandmother wouldn't recognize as food. There are a great many food-like items in the supermarket your ancestors wouldn't recognize as food... stay away from these."*
> **– Michael Pollan**

Negative Exposure

Fill your mind only with what you want in your life; only positive stimuli related to your goals and then by you will activate the power of the universal Law of Correspondence. The Law of Correspondence states that *the predominant thoughts held in your mind will soon be reflected in your outer life.* Your outer life is simply a mirror of what is going on inside of you in your *inner* life.

So by eliminating the negative influences and stimuli you're exposed to daily, you will create more positive, successful and joyous experiences in your everyday reality. Life is a mirror. What we think and feel about all day long, is what will then show up in our outside world. Everything first begins within our minds, so by not feeding it with negative information and influences we are much more likely to create a more positive lifestyle for ourselves.

> *"Be careful of the environment you choose for it will shape you, be careful the friends you choose for you will become like them."*
> **– W. Clement Stone**

Cut Out Snacking, Avoid Grazing

Snacking, particularly continual snacking sabotages all efforts of creating a leaner version of you. Every calorie adds up. Just keep your focus on eating a well-balanced, highly nutritious moderate sized meal *around every four hours.* The only snack that you should ever consider and incorporate would be a high quality, lean protein snack in the evening such as a protein and water shake, low-fat natural yoghurt or piece of lean meat, poultry, fish in order to prevent you from falling into a harmful state of deep physical hunger.

> *"Eat to live, don't live to eat."*
> **– Benjamin Franklin**

Binge Drinking

You already know the detrimental effects of alcohol on weight loss and overall health so avoid any kind of over-indulgence, especially binge drinking.

> *"First we form habits, then they form us. Conquer your bad habits or they will conquer you."*
> **– Rob Gilbert**

Sneaking in Empty Calories

These are the things we tend to overlook like: cream, sugar, syrups in your tea or coffees, soft drinks, cooking using more oil than required. They provide us with little in terms of nutritional value but load our bodies with extra calories.

Take my mum as an example of how easily this happens. My mum enjoys a cup of tea at different times throughout her day: her work break, when she visits a friend or family member's house or while she's relaxing back at the house after a long day at work watching the television. However, she sneaks in these empty excess calories by having a few biscuits, chocolates, a slice of cake, or any other form of processed foods that come out of a tin, box, wrapper or packet. At the time she may not consider the effect of a couple of chocolate digestives, but if we *add up* all these processed little treats we might be quite shocked by the additional non-nutritional calories. If these were replaced with fruits, lean proteins and vegetables my mum would be in top shape all year round.

If this is you, make sure that when you're offered the biscuit tray that you politely decline. You can choose enjoying the moment on a short term basis, or looking great on a long term basis, but you cannot choose both. That choice I'll have to leave with you.

> *"If you are going to achieve excellence in big things, you develop the habit in little matters. Excellence is not an exception, it is a prevailing attitude."*
> **– Colin Powell**

Mindless and Emotional Eating

Mindless eating is the act of *eating without being fully aware of what we're doing,* and often when we're not even hungry. Emotional eating (as discussed) is reactive eating to emotional stress. *Awareness* is the key to changing both of these behaviours.

> *"We are what we repeatedly do. Excellence, then, is not an act, but a habit."*
> **– Aristotle**

Divorce with the Habits that Hold You Back

> *"It is easier to prevent bad habits than to break them."*
> **– Benjamin Franklin**

Summary:

The One Month Challenge:

- Take one positive habit from those outlined in this chapter and discipline yourself to repeat it each and every single day for the entire month until it becomes second nature and natural to you. Set the habit you're going to consistently put into action as a goal on your monthly exercise calendar and follow it through day after day without fail for the entire month. At the end of the month, once you have successfully completed the challenge, you will have developed the muscle memory required to live out this new pattern in your life without even expending energy or conscious effort. It will now run for you on autopilot.

- Choose another positive habit for the following month to be repeated day in and day out until it becomes a natural part of your being. Repeat this process month after month, positive change after positive change until you have created an army of positive habits to go to work for you in your everyday routine and bring about excellent results.

- Take one negative habit from the list above that you recognise you're guilty of in your current routine and set the goal on your monthly exercise calendar to work to refrain from engaging in this behaviour for the entire month. At the end of the month, once you have successfully completed this challenge, you will have removed this self-limiting behaviour from your habitual behaviour patterns and will be one giant step closer to having the leanest physique you desire for yourself.

- Choose another negative habit your guilty of engaging in from your current routine in life to refrain from engaging in, set it as a goal for the following month on your monthly exercise calendar and get through the month without engaging in this self-limiting behaviour. Repeat the process month after month, eliminating one negative habit at a time until you have the best physique and highest level of health possible for yourself.

"We first make our habits, and then our habits make us."
– John Dryden

-9-

Strategies

Incorporate Winning Systems

In order to succeed in maintaining a lean, well defined physical appearance and a high degree of overall health, wellbeing and vitality, you will need to create your own daily systems that will positively promote these effects. Eliminate the things that don't work and keep the things that do.

Complete Kitchen Over-haul

Take an honest look at your eating and drinking patterns and you'll see the weaknesses and bad habits more clearly: eating the wrong things at weekends, lots of processed foods for example. There are many reasons that our households have a tendency to contain processed, junk foods or we choose to undo our good work with weekend pig-outs. We usually know when something's bad for us, but it's easy to find excuses.

We forget that actually *we are in control*. We can control what comes into our houses and therefore our kitchens and our mouths. We need to create the environment that mirrors that healthy image we desire. *It begins and ends in your kitchen*. The content stored in your cupboards, fridge and freezer will eventually create and define the shape of your physical appearance.

If you haven't already reached your ideal body weight and physique, maybe it's time for a complete kitchen overhaul. Go through all your cupboards, drawers, shelves, freezer, fridge and any other areas around your house that you may use to store any kind of food or drink and to throw any sugary, processed, junk foods away. Don't think, don't hesitate, simply take any food that is not whole, organic or fresh and discard it. Or if throwing away food is not in your nature or seems wasteful, then give it away to someone else who will appreciate it.

Now organise your kitchen in your own way to promote any of your new healthy eating and living habits that you've learned throughout this book. Stock up on green tea bags in your tea box, fill up your spice rack with metabolism boosting, health promoting spices, organise all your knives, kitchen essentials, food storage containers, create space in the fridge to store all your freshly chopped vegetables, place a fruit bowl on the table Use all your creativity in order to set yourself up for success in your new lifestyle habits and burn the self-limiting old ways of the past behind you. Do whatever is necessary in order to make sure that your kitchen fully represents the person you are now becoming.

Morning Weigh-ins

First thing in the morning, even before you jump in the shower, head straight for the bathroom and jump on the scales wearing only your underwear. During this time your body will be in a slightly dehydrated state. By checking your exact weight on a digital scale this time every day, you will keep your weigh-in circumstances consistent and therefore will be able to take the most accurate measurement of whether or not you're making progress in your weight loss efforts. If you manage to go to sleep at the end of each day in a slight state of negative energy balance, you should notice a slight reduction in your weight every day.

If you notice the weight slowly creeping back on, don't panic, simply reduce your portions and make the extra efforts to restore the slight state of negative energy balance that's essential for weight loss.

Fasted Morning Cardio

When you wake up, your body is in a *fasted state,* having not eaten since the night before. Therefore, if you exercise or expend a large amount of energy in this fasted state, your body will have to use its fat reserves. Fasted cardiovascular exercise is most commonly used by the more serious fitness enthusiasts. The exercise does not have to be of high intensity; moderate pace, longer, steady, continuous movement seems to work best.

Make sure the exercise sessions last a minimum of thirty minutes, up to an hour for optimal results. I also encourage you to consider a good natural fat burning supplement on your empty stomach to increase endurance and greatly enhance overall fat burning effects. Choose a cup of green tea, normal tea or coffee. You might also combine this by listening to motivational or inspirational audio tracks.

There are many different forms of moderate cardiovascular exercise to choose such as a fast morning walk, a light jog, a pool lane session or a cycle around your town.

Winning Shopping Habits

The art of war states that *every battle is won or lost before it's ever fought.* The *preparation before* any endeavour determines the results. Start the battle for a better physique with your shopping. See the guidelines earlier about only bringing into your home what you want to eat in order to win the war. Remember my advice to avoid the central aisles.

"Cultivate only the habits that you are willing shall master you."
– Elbert Hubbard

The Ultimate Weight Loss Pot

If there is a shortcut to natural, effortless loss of weight and body fat on a daily basis, then **this is it.** What you have to do is, buy yourself a slow cooking pot. You can get a great quality, large one for as little as £20. The idea is to buy a mixture of fresh spices, herbs, vegetables and a lean source of high quality protein. You would then roughly chop up all your ingredients and throw them into your slow cooking pot with a little water, stock and seasoning of your choice.

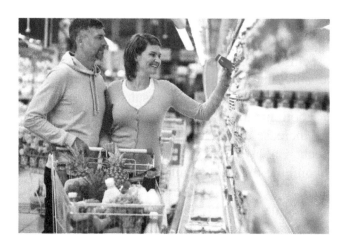

Turn the cooker on to heat, place the lid on the top and then leave it to cook out for about three or four hours on a high heat or between five and nine hours on a lower heat until all your vegetables and protein is thoroughly cooked. You would then just ladle your meal from the pot into a bowl and enjoy your meal.

This is possibly the most nutritious way to cook your meals. None of the essential nutrients will be lost in the cooking process. You may choose any fresh spices or vegetables that you like, and a lean source of protein could vary from fresh fish, lean cuts of meat, poultry, or tofu. The key is to ensure that only spices, vegetables and quality protein make it into your pot, by keeping out the starchy carbohydrates such as potatoes, rice, pasta, etc.; you will be ensuring that you end each of your days in a fat burning state

In order to make the sauce tasty, always add in stock cubes to match whatever lean source of protein you choose. For example, fish stock would go with haddock, vegetable stock with tofu and chicken stock if using chicken. Also consider including other ingredients such as tinned tomatoes, tomato puree, gravy mix or any other low-fat seasoning. If you don't have the time to wait around for three hours before your evening meal, consider putting your pot on to cook much earlier in your day, for example, before you leave for work.

Just make sure that you put your cooking temperature on your slow cooking pot to moderate or low, rather than high, so that it will cook out nicely over five, seven or even nine hours while you're busy labouring away at work that day. By making this highly nutritious, fresh produce 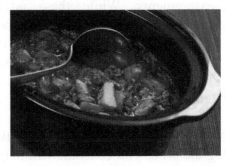 only, pot meals a part of your everyday routine, varying the combination and meals that you make, you will naturally assist weight loss. **Invest around £20 in a slow cooking pot and transform your physique.**

Body Composition Measurements

Weight and body composition are not the same thing. Weight might be made up of high levels of lean muscle and low levels of body fat, or low levels of lean muscle and excess body fat. Two people may weigh the same but look completely different, one fit and athletic; the other unfit and heavy-looking. The determining factor is their *body composition*. Body composition is the percentage of lean muscle to body fat tissue. This is determined by what we eat.

Naturally the weight of bones, water, organs and tissues are not under our control. But what we can control through action is this percentage of lean tissue to body fat. As you begin this journey you will see changes in your physical appearance from increasing the percentage of lean mass and reducing the percentage of body fat.

We can measure and track these results, for example using a body composition scale at a local gym or health club. Measurements are taken and you have a record that you can use for comparison as the weeks progress.

There are other ways to take measurements like skin fold callipers, Bioelectrical Impedance scales and hand grips; as well as more expensive equipment and methods used by health professionals and doctors. These include underwater weighing and x-ray scan measurements. While these advanced methods measure body composition directly, even using the basics such as viewing yourself in the mirror or receiving positive comments on your physique from others will be great indicators of your progress.

Make Yourself Accountable

Keep a food diary if it will help. Investing a few minutes each day to log the foods you consume will help provide focus and highlight bad habits. The very act of writing down on paper what you are eating, instantly makes you more accountable for your actions. Take control of what you feed yourself every day and align it with what the person with the body you're trying to achieve, would choose to eat.

Consider Personal Training

If you are struggling to follow these simple practical actions, *particularly exercise*, personal training may be an option for you. Although this book was initially created with the idea that anybody reading it could put it into action, I am aware that some of you are not as motivated to get down to the gym or stick to rigorous exercise regimes on your own.

You can find personal trainers offered through health clubs, community gyms and online but make sure you do your research. Check out all the trainer profiles, watch them in action training one of their clients or visit their website in order to gain an idea of how each trainer approaches their work and if you feel you would be comfortable spending a few hours a week in their company.

Look for someone of high character, a positive personality, open, caring and professional. If your intuition pulls you towards a particular trainer, then give them a call, send them an email or approach them in the gym and ask them nicely if you could book a consultation with them. Booking a consultation is essential before deciding if you want to invest your money, time and energy into a long term commitment with somebody. During a consultation, you would just have a short, brief, friendly conversation to find out about what they have to offer you and how they will help you to achieve your goals. Let them know a bit about your situation and lifestyle, and then together work out the best approach for you and get started.

Personal Visual Assessments

Results are a wonderful motivator and you can keep yourself on track or inspire others with photographs. Take photos of your body every week to see the changes for yourself. Many people who achieve astonishing results in their weight and fat loss efforts regret not taking before and after photos. When you feel you still have a long way to go, use the photos to show you how far you've come.

Some pointers:

1. Wearing a small pair of shorts (men) or a swimsuit (women), stand beside a long mirror.
2. Set up your camera about 5 – 7 feet away from yourself so that it can capture your whole body from head to toe.
3. Make sure that the room is well lit and that you use the highest quality camera settings.
4. Set a countdown timer on your camera to take the photo and make sure you take four photographs each week when you're taking your progress photos. One of the front side of your body. One of the left side of your body. One of the back side of your body. One of the right side of your body.
5. Every week, at the same time, in the same clothing, and using all the same camera settings, repeat the exact same four photos. File your photos on a folder in your computer or print them out on paper and keep them in a folder somewhere. Remember to log the date or week on each one.
6. After being consistent in your efforts in getting lean and losing weight for over four weeks, begin to lay out all the photos week by week, side by side. View your progress. If you're making slow, steady progress then keep doing what you are doing – well done. If you're no longer making any progress or even starting to gain a little more weight again, either increase your weekly exercise output, reduce your daily calorie intake from your meals or a

combination of both in order to signal your body to lose more weight and burn off body fat.

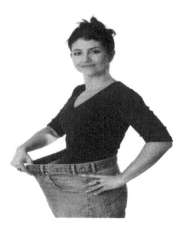

Eating Out Techniques and Tips

If you like to regularly eat in restaurants, you could be cancelling out your weight loss efforts so here are some things to consider and ways you can still enjoy this from time to time. The first thing you need to be aware of are the *portion sizes*. Restaurants tend to serve larger portions as well as offering more courses than you might be used to at home. This can create a massive caloric overload and overeating can be harmful to your body.

You can take control of this in a number of ways. You can restrict yourself by not having a starter or dessert or on special occasions consider sharing. A small bowl of fresh fruit salad would be best option if you absolutely must have dessert. If you choose to have a starter, choose a fresh low-fat soup or salad, these are very low in calories, yet highly nutritious and will ensure that you're satisfied after you've finished your main course.

Pass on the bread basket and stick with the side salad. Any dishes you order that come with bread, potatoes or chips, politely ask the waiter or waitress in advance if you can swap these starchy carbohydrates for a mixture of fresh vegetables or salad instead.

Don't worry; they get this request all the time. Stay focused on your goals and request lower calorie alternatives. When it's time to choose your main course, it helps to have a general understanding of cooking when reading the menu. Make all your choices with foods containing these key words in them; *grilled, baked, broiled, steamed or poached.*

If you're unsure of a specific description beside one of the choices, ask the waiting staff. If you want to wine and dine at restaurants regularly, make yourself familiar with these words and stay clear of them; *fried, crispy, battered, buttered, breaded, creamy, cheesy, deep-fried* as these will be high in fat and calories.

If you're eating at work then also think about how to avoid long-term issues associated with this. So for example if the canteen at your work serves a high calorie selection of fast foods and has a very limited selection of low calorie, highly nutritious alternatives then consider packing your own lunches or snacks with you to the workplace and avoid becoming a victim of your environment.

Whenever you are eating anywhere away from your own kitchen, take the time to thoroughly consider the choices you have, and choose the foods that your body will be thanking you for later.

The Sunday Ritual

Do you have a very busy working schedule? No time to spend cooking highly nutritious meals every day? Never at home to eat? The Sunday Ritual could be the optimal solution for you and your physique goals. The Sunday Ritual is a system that you can incorporate into your life to save time, money and allows you to control your eating schedule, what you eat and portion sizes.

To carry out The Sunday Ritual, select a day and time during the week where you have a spare one or two hours of solid, uninterrupted time. Sunday evening is a popular choice, hence its name: The Sunday Ritual. This is when you will prepare yourself for the week ahead. It only takes around two hours and saves you far more. **Below are the stages of The Sunday Ritual:**

First stage:

Sit down, think about the week ahead and then write down all the foods that you will need to purchase on the shopping trip for all the meals you want to eat each day for the following week.

Second stage:

Once you have a rough general idea of the type of meals you will be eating, visit your local supermarket, butchers, fishmongers or grocery shop and buy all the fresh, whole, nutrient dense foods and spices that you will need in order to prepare and cook your meals.

Third stage:

Once you get home from your shopping trip, it's now time to prepare and cook these meals in advance for the following week, organise them into meal containers, allow them to chill and put them away into your fridge until required for use. Then, simply microwave or reheat them thoroughly at meal times to enjoy them throughout the week. If you want to eat more fresh foods like salad you might want to make this ritual more frequent, perhaps several times a week; adapt according to your needs.

You want your meals to be as fresh as possible yet save yourself as much time in the kitchen as possible. I recommend two or three smaller full meal preparation days of around one hour each. Each week, or fortnight, consider reducing portion sizes. Your body will soon adapt and no longer require the same quantity of food to be satisfied and function optimally. Your stomach will shrink very gradually in a very healthy and natural manner. The key is not to rush this process, but gradually transform into a smaller version of yourself.

In the process of applying The Sunday Ritual into your routine, you will quickly develop and improve your cooking skills, food education, your self-discipline and organisational skills.

Into Action

(1) After buying your shopping, unpack foods into your cupboards and fridge. Keep out the food that you will be cooking for your busy workweek ahead. Peel, slice, or chop up any your fresh foods to be cooked.

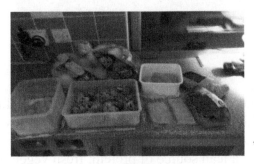

Prepare

(2) Cook off all your lean meats, fish, poultry, tofu, fresh vegetables, starchy carbohydrates etc. Then once they are cooked, leave your food out at room temperature or run under cold water to chill.

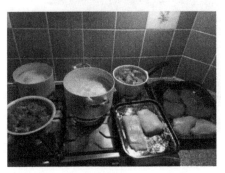

Cook

(3) Lay out all of your food storage containers on the counter ready to make up your own fresh, highly nutritious meals once your food has been cooked and chilled.

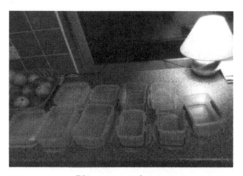

Your containers

(4) Once your cooked food has been thoroughly chilled, make up your meals in the containers. You are in full control of your portion sizes. Try to ensure that your meals are *well balanced,* containing a lean source of protein, fresh vegetables, and if you like, also some high quality starchy carbohydrates such as whole-grain rice or sweet potatoes. Also consider a low-fat homemade fresh sauce for taste.

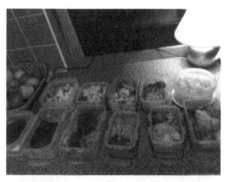

All boxed up and ready to chill

(5) Once you have made up your meals, store them away neatly in the fridge ready to be heated up in the microwave during your busy working schedule ahead. Make sure you do not cook too many meals so that they will not be fresh when it's time to eat

162

them, consider doing this ritual every three or four days if you can.

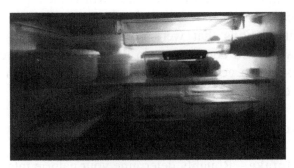

Chilled ready for use

(6) Have fun with this. Always strive to improve your current cooking skills and inventory. Experiment with different foods, tastes and combinations. Always use the highest quality, nutrient dense, low calorie foods.

Bulk Buying, Money Saving, Goal Achieving

To ensure that you always have high quality sources of fresh lean protein consider buying your protein foods from organic local sources such as butchers, fresh fish shops and larger food stores in bulk quantity then freeze them for later use. When you buy large amounts of lean produce from these sources they tend to give you a higher rate of discount the more you purchase. You could also consider cooking meals in bulk and freezing them.

Keep Yourself Busy

The more things you have going on in your life, the less you will focus on food. Food will become an enjoyable necessity but it will not control you.

Overcoming Plateaus

Most of us start out really well but there will come a point when you reach a plateau; you seem to be staying in the same place even if you continue with actions that were effective initially. As explained, insanity is when you continue to do the same things, over and over again, yet expect to get different results. So when this happens you need to make further changes.

Consider/Adjust the following factors:

1. **Food Intake** – Roughly determine your calorie intake and your portion size and ensure you have not unconsciously increased it. Are you snacking? Have you been eating foods high in sugar? If your weight loss is no longer decreasing each morning when you hop on the scales, take a look back over your days and find out where you can cut back a little here and there.

2. **Food Quality** – How high in nutrients and low in calories are the foods that make up each meal throughout your day? Does your diet consist mainly of lean proteins and fresh vegetables?

3. **Exercise Quality** – Are you focusing on *the quality* of your cardiovascular exercise, resistance training, weight training, cycling, walking, whatever the type of movement you engage in? How long, how hard, how fast, or how much effort are you putting into each of these sessions? If you feel you are no longer putting in as much as you once did, you will not get out as much as you once got out. Maybe you need to increase the duration of your light jog on the treadmill by another ten minutes each session, you may have to lift one stage higher in the weight room or you even swim another ten lengths in the pool. Whatever your current output, consider increasing it a little extra in order to get more return on your energy in order

to continue seeing improvements in your weight loss and overall physique.

4. **Exercise Quantity** – *How often* are you exercising each week? You may need to schedule another hour or two of exercise into your monthly exercise calendar in order to continue to lose weight, tone yourself up and burn away that unwanted body fat.

Strategies and Changes

Action-plan/ implementation

Chosen Strategy	How it can benefit my health, weight loss, fat loss, muscle building or performance level	When to consume in my current routine	Implemented into my routine to accelerate my progress towards my goals. ☑
			☐
			☐
			☐
			☐

-10-

Cooking and Recipes

Develop your Cooking Skills

Aside from being a personal trainer and a nightclub doorman, I've also spent six years in a kitchen. I worked as a chef creating all kinds of well-known dishes from all over the world. Some examples include: lasagnes, spaghetti dishes, penne dishes, curries, biryanis, chilli con carnies, famous chicken dishes, stir fries, stews, spiced rice dishes, soups, salads and a variety of popular fresh fish such as lemon sole, haddock, sea bass, salmon, scallops and mussels. My focus has always been on **healthy eating.**

Over this period of my life I developed a strong passion and understanding of real, fresh, clean, natural produce and how to best prepare, cook and combine these whole, single ingredient foods into tasty, nutritious dishes. In this chapter, I'll hand over a few basic essential tips that will maximise your time spent in the kitchen.

"Let food be thy medicine and medicine be thy food."
– Hippocrates

Kitchen Essentials

Getting started this is what you need:

Appliances:

- Oven
- Stove

- Microwave (optional)
- Fridge. Freezer
- Hand Blender (optional)
- Steamer (optional)
- Kettle

Essentials:

- Chopping board
- Small knife
- Chef's chopping knife
- Serrated carving knife
- Peeler
- Hand whisk
- Wooden cooking spoons
- Hot Food Flipper/Lifter Spatula
- Plastic mixing bowl
- Cooking trays
- Non-stick pans
- Pots
- Colander/Strainer
- Can opener
- Plastic/Glass food storage containers
- Protein Shaker(s) (optional)
- Grater, Rolling Pin, Scissors, Potato masher (optional)

The above appliances and tools will help you prepare and cook at the highest level. I have kept things very simple; the fundamentals are all you need.

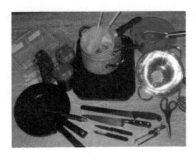

Always Cook Low Fat

Always make sure that you cook using the *minimal amount* of oil or fat required to reduce the total calorie count and fat content. The right amount is just enough to heat the food and prevent it from sticking to the bottom of the pot or pan. The most effective way to ensure this is to *spray* cooking oil rather than pour it.

There are a few cooking oils that I recommend: extra-virgin olive oil makes a very light salad drizzle and can be used when cooking foods at **lower heats** as it tends to burn when used to cook at higher temperatures. Walnut oil can also be used as a very light salad dressing. Coconut oil should be used while cooking at **higher heats** in small amounts in order to provide you with essential good fats, and provide a slight thermic effect that helps to minimise overall calorie count.

Refrain from using vegetable, rapeseed, canola and corn oils as when taken frequently in excess they can cause a variety of health issues, such as chronic inflammation, arthritis, diabetes, heart disease and other potential problems due to an imbalance of omega-6 fats and too little omega-3 fats.

Avoid all the high fat cooking methods such as deep frying, using more oil than necessary while pan frying and topping cooked food with butter for flavouring. Focus on cooking your food using minimal or zero fat cooking methods such as oven roasting, baking, oven grilling, boiling, steaming, poaching, light pan frying using a few light sprays of olive or coconut oil. The goal should be to get your food cooked using a little oil as possible, using the most basic and natural traditional cooking methods available to us.

"Don't dig your grave with your own knife and fork."
– English proverb

Building your Meals and Snacks

Were you paying attention earlier?
To maintain and build lean muscle tissue while burning body fat, there is a specific formula for every meal or snack. Each meal must contain? You're right: a high quality source of lean protein, low calorie, highly nutritious vegetables or fresh fruit and whole-grain carbohydrates in smaller amounts earlier in the day.

Always think protein, vegetables, fruits, starchy carbohydrates in that order. I have left the omega-3, healthy essential fats out here as you should be getting them along with the specific proteins, vegetables, fruit or supplements that you consume.

Spice It Up

Small quantities of different spices and herbs can benefit your health as well as add interesting flavours to meals. They can also provide a number of health benefits such as: fight infection, boost the immune system, reduce inflammation, prevent cancer, improve heart health, keep skin healthy, regulate the metabolism, detoxify the body, lose weight, strengthen bones, reduce stress, increase digestion, protect against dozens of dangerous diseases, cure colds, protect oral health, contribute to a healthy diet and balance the hormones in our body.

The trick is to enhance your meals with the spice that creates the greatest flavour, while providing necessary health benefits to suit your needs. Many spices also raise metabolism shortly after we eat so can aid weight loss.

"The doctor of the future will no longer treat the human frame with drugs, but rather will cure and prevent disease with nutrition."
– Thomas Edison

Examples of Spices:

- Ground Cinnamon
- Ground Nutmeg
- Ground Cardamom
- Ground Cumin
- Ground Ginger
- Ground Turmeric
- Ground Coriander
- Chinese Five Spice
- Paprika
- Chilli Power
- Chilli Seeds
- Black Pepper
- Cayenne Pepper

Fresh Spices:

- Fresh Garlic
- Fresh Chilli
- Fresh Ginger

Fresh Herbs:

- Parsley
- Coriander
- Basil
- Rosemary
- Thyme
- Oregano
- Tarragon

Choosing spices and understanding their benefits is a great way to enhance your cooking for your health and if this subject really captures your interest then be sure to do your research online or from a good book on spices.

Breakfast Ideas

Yes it is true: breakfast really is the most important meal of the day. By making sure that you feed yourself with the highest quality nutrients early in the morning you will kick-start your metabolism. Think of it like loading fuel into a race car before the race. The higher the quality of nutrients during this first meal, the greater your physical and mental performance over the course of the day.

There are three different options you can consider for breakfast: egg-based meals, fruit-based meals or oatmeal-based meals. I'll provide a basic sample recipe of each and some ingredients that you can incorporate into the meal to create it uniquely for your own needs and personal preferences.

Breakfast Ideas

Egg-based Breakfast Options:

1. **Omelette** (Serves 1)

    Ingredients:

    - 1 whole egg
    - 3 egg whites
    - Small splash of low-fat milk
    - Finely diced fresh spices of choice
    - Cooked and chopped vegetables of choice
    - Cooked and diced source of lean protein of choice (fish, chicken, beef, tofu, ham, etc.)
    - Spices and herbs of choice for taste. (Ground pepper, paprika, chilli powder, etc.)

Cooking Instructions:

1. Using a little coconut or olive oil, lightly coat a large non-stick frying pan on medium heat.
2. Add any fresh spices that you want to include such as garlic, chilli, ginger or diced onion and then sauté until lightly browned, stirring frequently.
3. Add cooked and diced fresh vegetables and choice of lean protein and sauté for 1 minute more.
4. Re-spray pan if needed and then add the mixture of egg whites, whole egg, spices or herbs that you have thoroughly whisked in a separate mixing bowl.
5. Cook until the top of the mixture begins to bubble and the bottom is golden brown.
6. Flip the omelette and cook the other side until golden brown.
7. Transfer the omelette to a plate.
8. Enjoy.

2. **Scramble** (Serves 1)

Ingredients:

- 1 whole egg
- 3 egg whites
- Small splash of low-fat milk
- Cooked and chopped fresh spices of choice
- Cooked and chopped fresh vegetables of choice
- Cooked and chopped fresh lean protein of choice
- Herbs and spices of choice for taste

Cooking Instructions:

1. Lightly coat a non-stick frying pan with coconut or olive oil spray on medium heat.
2. Add your fresh spices and lean protein of choice then sauté off until lightly browned.

3. Add your freshly chopped cooked vegetables and cook out for a few minutes more.
4. Remove cooked spices, vegetables and protein from pan into a separate bowl.
6. Re-spray the pan and then add your mixture of whole egg, egg whites, a splash of milk and your spices and herbs of choice that you have whisked in a separate mixing bowl.
7. Cook the egg mixture whole stirring constantly to break up the egg.
8. Once all egg mixture has been cooked, add spices, vegetables and protein mixture back into the pan and cook further for around 1 minute.
9. Transfer mixture to a plate.
10. Enjoy.

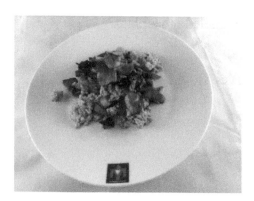

Salmon, spinach, red pepper, tomato and mushroom scramble

3. Frittata (Serves 1)

Ingredients:

- 2 whole eggs
- 3 egg whites
- Small splash of low-fat milk
- Fine diced fresh spices of choice

- Fine diced fresh vegetables of choice
- Fine diced lean protein of choice
- Spices and herbs of choice for taste.
- Low-fat feta cheese (crumbled) or buffalo mozzarella cheese (finely sliced) (optional)

Cooking Instructions:

1. Lightly coat a large non-stick frying pan with coconut or olive oil spray on medium heat.
2. Add fresh spices and lean protein of choice. Sauté until golden brown.
3. Add fresh vegetables of choice and cook for a further couple of minutes.
4. Evenly pour the egg mixture of whole eggs, egg whites, milk and spices that you have whisked together thoroughly in a separate mixing bowl over the ingredients in your pan.
5. Cook mixture on medium heat for a couple of minutes until the top begins to bubble.
6. Evenly spread a small amount of cheese over the top of your mixture and place the whole pan into the oven for a few minutes until the egg is cooked.
7. Transfer the mixture from the pan onto a plate.
8. Enjoy.

4. Breakfast Quiche (Serves 1)

Ingredients:

- 2 whole eggs
- 3 egg whites
- Small splash of low-fat milk
- Fresh herbs of choice finely diced
- Cooked lean protein of choice finely diced
- Cooked fresh vegetables of choice finely diced
- Spices and herbs of choice for taste

• Small amount of low-fat Swiss cheese (optional)

Cooking Instructions:

1. Preheat the oven to a moderate high heat.
2. Add all the ingredients into a blender.
3. Blend the mixture thoroughly until smooth consistency.
4. Lightly coat a non-stick muffin tray with coconut or olive oil spray.
5. Evenly distribute the mixture into each muffin cup, filling each half way.
6. Bake in oven until the egg is cooked all the way through (20 minutes approx.).
7. Remove muffin tray from oven, allow a minute to cool, use spoon to slide the quiches out of the muffin cups onto a plate.
8. Enjoy.

Fruit-based Breakfast Options:

1) Mixed Fruit Salad topped with yoghurt or protein mixture
(Serves 1)

Ingredients:

• 2+ different kinds of fresh fruit
• Low-fat natural yoghurt or flavoured whey protein whisked with small splash of milk or water
• Small drizzle of honey (optional)
• Ground Flaxseeds (optional)

Preparation Instructions:

1. Chop up your fruit into bite sized cubes or slices.
2. Mix the fruits together with ground flaxseed (optional) and place mixture into a bowl.

3. Top with a few spoons of low-fat natural yoghurt or flavoured whey protein mixture (chocolate/vanilla/strawberry, etc.).
4. Drizzle lightly with some pure honey (optional).

2. **Mixed berry salad topped with yoghurt or protein** mixture (Serves 1)

Ingredients:

- Blueberries, raspberries, strawberries, acai berries, blackberries or many other type of berries
- Low-fat natural yoghurt
- Flavoured whey protein whisked with splash of low-fat milk or water (strawberry/chocolate/vanilla etc.)
- Ground Flaxseed (optional)
- Honey (optional)
- Finely chopped fresh mint (optional)

Preparation Instructions:

1. Combine a mixture of different types of berries with ground flaxseed (optional) and fresh mint (optional).
2. Transfer mixture into a bowl and then top with low-fat natural yoghurt or flavoured protein mixture.
3. Lightly drizzle with honey (optional).
4. Enjoy.

3. **Mixed fruit and berry salad topped with yoghurt or protein mixture** (Serves 1)

Ingredients:

- 1+ different kinds of fresh fruit (diced or sliced)
- 1+ different kinds of berries
- Low-fat natural yoghurt or flavoured whey protein whisked with small splash of milk or water

- Small drizzle of honey (optional)
- Ground Flaxseeds (optional)
- Finely chopped fresh mint (optional)

Preparation Instructions:

1. Combine your mixture of fruit and berries with ground flaxseed (optional) and fresh mint (optional).
2. Transfer mixture into a bowl and then top with low-fat natural yoghurt or flavoured protein mixture.
3. Lightly drizzle with honey (optional).
4. Enjoy.

Oatmeal-based Breakfast Options

1) Oatmeal porridge with fruit and topped with yoghurt or protein mixture (Serves 1)

Ingredients:

- Whole Oats or oatmeal
- Water or green tea infused water
- 1 fresh fruit of choice (sliced or chopped)
- Low-fat natural yoghurt or flavoured whey protein whisked with a small splash of low-fat milk or water
- Ground Cinnamon or Ground Nutmeg (optional)
- Ground Flaxseed (optional)
- Small drizzle of honey (optional)

Cooking Instructions:

1. Bring water or green tea to the boil in a small pot on medium heat.
2. Add the oats and spice of choice (optional). Reduce heat to medium-low and simmer for 5 – 10 minutes until oats are cooked while stirring occasionally.

3. Remove pot from heat then mix in your chopped fruit and ground flaxseed (optional).
4. Transfer oats from pot into a bowl then top with low-fat yoghurt or protein mixture.
5. Lightly drizzle with honey (optional).
6. Enjoy.

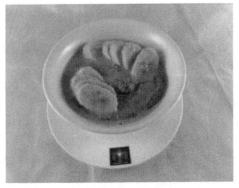

Banana, honey, cinnamon and vanilla protein oatmeal

Lunch Ideas

1) Mixed Salad (Serves 1)

Ingredients:

- Lettuce/mixed leaves/ spinach of choice (shredded/chopped)
- Raw vegetables & fruits of choice (peppers, tomatoes, cucumber, spring onion, red onion, carrots, celery, avocado, olives, etc.)
- Cooked vegetables of choice (e.g. broccoli, cauliflower, mushrooms, asparagus, courgettes, peppers, green beans, sugar snaps, peas, baby corn, beetroot, etc.)
- Fresh herbs and spices of choice finely chopped (e.g. coriander, basil, parsley, ginger, chilli, etc.)
- Cooked lean protein of choice (e.g. chicken, tuna, salmon, beef, gammon, egg, tofu, etc.)

- Ground Flaxseed (optional)
- Light salad dressing (walnut oil, extra virgin olive oil, balsamic vinegar, etc.)

Preparation Instructions:

1. Place your lean proteins on a baking tray, season with spices of your choice (optional), roast in the oven until cooked. Remove from oven and allow to cool at room temperature or using a chiller. Place into container and into fridge to be used in all your cold salad meals.
2. Take out cooked meat from fridge, slice into thin slices or cubes on a chopping board.
3. Shred or slice up your lettuce leaves, raw and/or cooked vegetables and fresh herbs and spices.
4. In a large mixing bowl, combine all ingredients with some ground flaxseed (optional) and then transfer into a bowl.
5. Lightly drizzle with salad dressing of choice
6. Enjoy.
   (Spinach, iceberg, baby gem, romaine, mixed leaves, other) buy fresh and slice up at home, avoid packaged versions if possible to maximize nutritional content and avoid any chemicals or toxins.)

2) Your Choice of oven roasted lean protein served with freshly cooked vegetables and topped with low-fat sauce (Serves 1)

Ingredients:

- Lean Protein of your choice (e.g. chicken breast, fresh fish, lean cuts of meat, tofu steak etc.)
- Mixture of fresh vegetables of your choice (e.g. broccoli, cauliflower, carrots, baby corn, peas, sugar snaps, green beans, sweet born, or roasted spices and vegetables such as ginger, chilli, peppers onions, courgettes, aubergines, mushrooms, etc.)

- Ground spices for seasoning (e.g. Cajun spices, Mexican spices, ground pepper, ground cumin, ground coriander, curry powder, etc.)
- Small amount of low-fat sauce of choice for taste (e.g. BBQ, sweet chilli, pesto, honey, or another type of sauce. (Ensure that you only use a small amount to add taste and keep calories count low.)

Cooking Instructions:

1. Lightly spray a non-stick frying pan with coconut or extra-virgin olive oil and bring to medium heat.
2. Add your lean protein of choice and season well a combination of ground spices of your choosing (e.g. Cajun spices, ginger, and coriander).
3. Lightly brown your protein on both sides, then place pan into oven on moderate heat or transfer onto a lightly sprayed baking tray and place into the oven until cooked (around 20 – 40 minutes).
4. Cook your mixed vegetables either by boiling in a pot, steaming in the steamer or lightly sprayed and roasted in the oven.
5. Once your vegetables and lean protein is cooked, transfer to a plate and top with a small amount of low-fat sauce for taste
6. Enjoy.

3. Whole-grain Salad Wrap (Serves 1)

Ingredients:

- 100% whole-grain tortilla
- Lettuce or salad leaves of choice (e.g. Romaine, iceberg, baby gem, mixed leaves, spinach, etc.)
- Cooked and sliced lean source of protein of choice (e.g. fresh fish, lean cuts of meat, chicken, turkey, eggs, tofu, etc.)

• Cooked and chopped vegetables of choice (e.g. peppers, tomatoes, cucumber, red onion, spring onion, carrots, etc.)
• Light amount of low-fat spread of choice for taste (optional) (e.g. low-fat Philadelphia cream cheese, low-fat Greek yoghurt, low-fat crème fraiche, salsa, etc.) You could also mix a choice of ground spice with your yoghurt or cheese for example, Cajun spiced yoghurt or chilli crème cheese
• Fresh spices of choice (optional) (e.g. shredded chilli, shredded ginger, etc.)
• Ground Flaxseed (optional)

Preparation Instructions:

1. Shred up all your protein, lettuce, vegetables and fresh spices (optional) of choice. Place them in a mixing bowl with ground flaxseed (optional) and thoroughly combine together.
2. Combine your low-fat spread with any ground spices of choice (optional) and then lightly spread one side of your tortilla.
3. Transfer the filling mixture from your mixing bowl onto the side of your tortilla that you have spread. Make sure you don't place too many contents into the wrap or it will not roll.
4. Firmly roll over your wrap to secure all the contents inside.
5. Slice the wrap in half using a serrated knife.
7. Enjoy.

4. Lettuce Wrap (Serves 1)

Ingredients:

• Iceberg lettuce
• Cooked and sliced lean source of protein of choice (e.g. fresh fish, lean cuts of meat, chicken, turkey, eggs, tofu, etc.)
• Cooked and chopped vegetables of choice (e.g. peppers, tomatoes, cucumber, red onion, spring onion, carrots, etc.)
• Light amount of low-fat spread of choice for taste (optional) (e.g. low-fat Philadelphia cream cheese, low-fat Greek

yoghurt, low-fat crème fraiche, salsa, etc.). You could also mix a choice of ground spice with your yoghurt or cheese for example, Cajun spiced yoghurt or chilli crème cheese)
- Fresh spices of choice (optional) (e.g. shredded chilli, shredded ginger, etc.)
- Ground Flaxseed (optional)

Preparation Instructions:

1. Shred up all your protein, lettuce, vegetables and fresh spices (optional) of choice. Place them in a mixing bowl with ground flaxseed (optional) and thoroughly combine together.
2. Combine your low-fat spread with any ground spices of choice (optional) and then lightly spread one side of your iceberg lettuce leaves (use a few layers of the larger outer leaves held firmly together).
3. Transfer the filling mixture from your mixing bowl onto the side of your lettuce that you have spread. Make sure you don't place too many contents into the wrap or it will not roll.
4. Firmly roll over your wrap to secure all the contents inside.
5. Slice the wrap in half using a serrated knife
6. Enjoy.

5. Spiced whole-grain rice with vegetables (Serves 1+)

Ingredients:

- 100% whole-grain rice (cooked and chilled)
- Finely diced cooked lean protein of choice (e.g. fresh fish, prawns, chicken, lean cuts of meat, tofu. etc.)
- Finely diced fresh spices of choice (chilli, garlic, ginger, etc.)
- Finely diced cooked vegetables of choice (e.g. mixed peppers, carrots, courgettes, onions, aubergines, green beans, baby corn, peas, spinach etc.)
- Roughly chopped fresh coriander (optional)

- Ground spices of choice (cinnamon, chilli powder, chilli flakes, paprika, pepper, coriander, ginger, cumin, curry powder, Piri Piri spice, turmeric or other spices may enjoy)
- A sauce or paste of your choice for taste (e.g. hot curry paste, sweet chili sauce, hot chilli sauce, tomato puree, soy sauce, BBQ sauce)
- Stock. Chicken, beef, fish or vegetable matching your choice of lean source of protein

Cooking Instructions:

1. Sauté diced fresh spices: garlic, chilli, ginger and onions until soft in a pan on moderate heat using a little coconut or extra-virgin olive oil spray.
2. Add mixture of ground spices and a little water. Simmer for 10 – 20 minutes until cooked and a thin paste.
3. Add diced cooked protein and vegetables and cook out for five minutes.
4. Add in your cooked, strained rice and sauce or paste for taste. Cook for 3 – 5 minutes, stirring frequently.
5. Transfer your spicy rice onto plate and top with fresh chopped ground coriander (optional).
6. Enjoy.

Evening Meal Ideas

1) Your Choice of oven roasted lean protein served with freshly cooked vegetables and topped with low-fat sauce (Serves 1)

Ingredients:

- Lean protein of your choice (e.g. chicken breast, fresh fish, lean cuts of meat, tofu steak etc.)
- Mixture of fresh vegetables of your choice (e.g. broccoli, cauliflower, carrots, baby corn, peas, sugar snaps, green beans, sweet born, or roasted spices and vegetables such as

ginger, chilli, peppers onions, courgettes, aubergines, mushrooms, etc.)
- Ground spices for seasoning (e.g. Cajun spices, Mexican spices, ground pepper, ground cumin, ground coriander, curry powder, etc.)
- Small amount of low-fat sauce of choice for taste (e.g. BBQ, sweet chilli, pesto, honey, or another type of sauce. (Ensure that you only use a small amount to add taste and keep calories count low)

Cooking Instructions:

1. Lightly spray a non-stick frying pan with coconut or extra-virgin olive oil and bring to medium heat.
2. Add your lean protein of choice and season well a combination of ground spices of your choosing (e.g. Cajun spices, ginger, and coriander).
3. Lightly brown your protein on both sides, then place pan into oven on moderate heat or transfer onto a lightly sprayed baking tray and place into the oven until cooked (around 20 – 40 minutes).
4. Cook your mixed vegetables either by boiling in a pot, steaming in the steamer or lightly sprayed and roasted in the oven.
5. Once your vegetables and lean protein is cooked, transfer to a plate and top with a small amount of low-fat sauce for taste.
6. Enjoy.
7. Freshly prepare mixed salad served with lean protein and a light salad dressing (Serves 1)

2) Your Choice of oven roasted lean protein served on a fresh vegetable salad. (Serves 1)

Ingredients:

- Lean protein of choice (e.g. fresh fish, lean cut of meat, chicken, turkey, tofu, etc.)
- Lettuce or salad leaves of choice (e.g. iceberg lettuce, romaine lettuce, baby-gem lettuce, mixed leaves etc.)
- Mixture of freshly chopped vegetables of choice (e.g. mixed peppers, carrots, cucumber, tomatoes, red onion, spring onion, or cooked and chilled asparagus, broccoli, green beans, baby corn, etc.)
- Fresh spices of choice (optional) (e.g. sliced ginger, chilli, etc.)
- Fresh herbs of choice (optional) (e.g. coriander, basil, parsley, etc.)
- Ground spices of choice to for seasoning (e.g. Mexican spice, Cajun spices, chilli powder, curry powder, ground cumin, ground coriander, etc.)
- Ground Flaxseeds (optional)
- Low-fat salad dressing of choice (optional) (e.g. extra-virgin olive oil, balsamic vinegar, walnut oil, etc.)

Preparation and Cooking Instructions:

1. Lightly coat a non-stick frying pan with coconut oil or olive oil. Brown off both sides of your lean protein on a medium heat with all the spices you choice to season it with of your own choice (e.g. 1 breast of chicken, seasoned with Mexican spices, a little ground cumin and a little ground coriander).
2. Once your protein has been browned off on both sides, place the pan into the oven on a moderate heat for 20 – 30 minutes until cooked. You could similarly place the protein onto a lightly greased baking tray and put that into the oven also.

3. While your protein is roasting in the oven, shred up all your lettuce and chop up all your fresh spices, vegetables and herbs. Combine them all together in a mixing bowl with ground flaxseed (optional) and a light drizzle of low-fat salad dressing of choice for taste.
4. Once your protein has been cooked, remove from the oven, and cut into fine slices on a chopping board.
5. Transfer your mixed salad onto a plate and then place the cooked protein on top.
6. Enjoy.

3) Fresh homemade curry served with whole-grain rice
(Serves 1+)

Ingredients:

- 100% Whole-grain rice
- Fresh garlic cloves, fresh chilli, fresh ginger (finely diced)
- Lean protein of choice (e.g. chicken, turkey, lean cuts of meat, tofu, and sweet potato). (Cut into cubes)
- Fresh vegetables of choice (e.g. mixed peppers, celery, onions, green beans, carrots, broccoli, cauliflower, baby corn, courgettes, aubergines, etc.)
- Ground Spices: curry powder, garam masala, ground turmeric, ground ginger, ground coriander, chilli powder, paprika. You may add some others as required.
- Chicken, beef or vegetable stock. Whatever type of lean protein you are making, use the same stock to complement it. For example if you're making a chicken curry, use chicken stock, if tofu or sweet potato curry, use vegetable stock and so on)
- Freshly chopped tomatoes or tinned tomatoes
- Tomato puree or paste
- Fresh coriander
- Low-fat natural Greek yoghurt

Cooking Instructions:

1. To cook your rice, bring a pot of water to boil then add the rice. Leave your rice to cook for around 20 – 30 minutes while you prepare the rest of your meal.
2. In a pot sauté off your finely diced fresh chillies, onions, garlic, ginger using a little coconut or extra virgin olive oil on a medium heat.
3. Once fresh spices are cooked, add in a small equal amount of your ground spices: Curry powder, garam masala, ground coriander, ground cumin, chilli powder/paprika and any others you want to include.
4. Add a tiny pinch of turmeric.
5. Reduce heat to medium/low and simmer these spices for around 20 – 30 minutes until thoroughly cooked out. Add a little water whenever the liquid in the pan reduces right down.
6. Add your freshly chopped tomatoes or tinned tomatoes, tomato paste and some freshly chopped coriander to your cooked spices and simmer for 5 – 10 minutes on medium heat.
7. Use a blender to puree this into a fine sauce (optional).
8. Put aside this pan of sauce for later.
9. In a separate pot, lightly spray using coconut oil or extra-virgin olive oil and sauté off raw diced lean protein of choice until lightly browned all over on the outside.
10. Add your roughly chopped fresh spices and vegetables of choice and sauté off for a few minutes.
11. Once your protein and vegetables have been lightly cooked on the outside, pour your curry sauce mixture into this pot and simmer on a moderate heat for 10 – 30 minutes until the protein and vegetables are thoroughly cooked.
12. Remove pot from the heat then add a couple spoons of low-fat natural yoghurt and some freshly chopped coriander. Make sure you remove the pot from the heat so that when you add the yoghurt to the sauce it will not split.
13. Drain your rice well using a colander, and then leave it to stand for around three minutes.

14. Transfer the rice onto a plate, and then ladle your curry over the top.
15. Enjoy.

4) Fresh homemade chilli con carne served with whole-grain rice
(Serves 1+)

Ingredients:

- 100% whole-grain rice
- Beef or Quorn mince
- Finely diced fresh spices: garlic gloves, chillies, ginger, onions
- Finely diced fresh vegetables: carrots, red peppers, celery, onions
- Tinned cooked red kidney beans
- Ground spices: chilli powder/paprika, chilli flakes, cinnamon, ground pepper, ground cumin, ground ginger. (You may add other spices as required)
- Freshly chopped tomatoes or tinned tomatoes
- Tomato puree or tomato paste
- Beef or vegetable stock
- Freshly chopped coriander (optional)
- Small amount of freshly grated cheddar cheese for presentation only (optional)

Cooking Instructions:

1. Lightly spray a pot with coconut or extra-virgin olive oil and heat on a moderate heat.
2. Add your diced fresh garlic, ginger, onions and chillies and sauté for a few minutes until softened.
3. Add beef or Quorn mince to the pot and cook off this mince in its own juices using a wooden spoon to break up any chunks of mince until lightly browned.

4. Add in all your ground spices, freshly chopped or tinned tomatoes, tomato puree, stock and a little water if required.
5. Reduce the heat to moderate/low and simmer for around 1 hour, stirring frequently and adding any more water if required until the mixture is rich and thickened.
6. To cook your rice, bring a pot of water to boil then add the rice. Leave your rice to cook for around 20 – 30 minutes while you prepare the rest of your meal.
7. Add in your strained kidney beans and freshly chopped coriander and cook gently for a further ten minutes, adding any extra seasoning if necessary.
8. Drain your rice well using a colander, and then leave it to stand for around three minutes.
9. Transfer the rice onto a plate, and then ladle your chili over the top.
10. Enjoy.

5) Fresh homemade protein and vegetable stir-fry with noodles
(Optional) (Serves 1+)

Ingredients:

- Fresh Spices: ginger, chilli, garlic (finely chopped)
- Onion of choice (e.g. white, red or spring onion) (optional)
- Chopped lean protein source of choice (e.g. prawns, chicken, lean cuts of meat, tofu, etc.)
- Fresh vegetables of choice (e.g. cooked broccoli, baby corn, cauliflower, carrots green beans or raw mixed peppers, celery, mushrooms, etc.)
- Noodles
- Soy sauce
- Oyster sauce
- Stock: use the same stock as the choice of protein you use. e.g. fish stock if you use prawns, or veg stock if you use tofu
- Ground spices of choice (e.g. ginger, chilli, pepper, coriander, chilli flakes, etc.) (optional)

• Fresh coriander (optional)

Cooking Instructions:

1. To prepare your noodles (if you decide to include them in this meal) place them in a mixing bowl or pot and cover with boiling water. Leave to sit for around 10 minutes until cooked. Once cooked, strain them in a colander and then leave sitting nearby for later.
2. In a large frying pan (wok style if possible), lightly spray with coconut or extra-virgin olive oil and add finely chopped fresh spices: garlic, chilli, ginger with your finely chopped onion of choice (optional). Cook until soft on a medium heat.
3. Add in your chopped raw lean protein of choice and cook until browned on all sides.
4. Add in a little stock, as well as a couple spoons each of soy and oyster sauce. Simmer for five minutes to cook protein and sauce.
5. Add in ground spices of choice for taste and any raw or cooked vegetables you want to include. Allow to simmer for a few minutes.
6. Add your cooked, strained noodles (optional) and freshly chopped coriander (optional) and simmer for 3 – 5 minutes while mixing thoroughly using a spoon.
7. Transfer to a plate.
8. Enjoy.

Snack Ideas

1. Whole fresh fruit
2. Low-fat natural Greek style yoghurt
3. Fresh berries
4. Flavoured whey protein powder + water shake
5. Flavoured whey protein + low-fat milk or water mixture
6. High quality lean protein bar
7. Mixed vegetable salad

8. Cooked or chilled lean source of protein
9. Combination of any of the above.

Examples:

• Sliced fresh fruit + low-fat natural yoghurt.
• Mixed fresh berries + flavoured whey protein mixture.
• Fresh vegetable salad + chilled sliced chicken/tuna/egg.

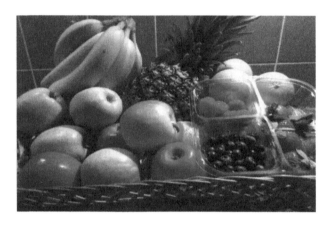

"The healthy man is the thin man. But you don't need to go hungry for it: Remove the flours, starches and sugars; that's all."
    – Samael Aun Weor

-11-

The System

Organise All your Knowledge into Practical Plans of Action

In order to lose a massive amount of body weight and fat and bring out the best in your physical shape, tone and definition, your job is to now take everything you have learned, from each area of this book and *combine them together* so that they work in perfect harmony and synergy with each other.

When you eat the right foods, at the right times, in the right amounts, you will begin to lose weight. If you also exercise a few days of the week, you will lose more weight and look even better in a much shorter period of time. Now combine these changes with a more positive way of thinking, introduce a few powerful habits, a strategy, better cooking skills, some supplements and you will have the ultimate blend; **you will give yourself the power for positive change in your life and the results will be astonishing.**

Within days, you'll notice people around you pointing out how they feel you've changed, how you look healthier, more vibrant, optimistic and happy with yourself. So here's how you use The System.

Part 1 – Your Diet

There are **two goals** that you must and absolutely need to hit in order to succeed in the eating part of this system:

The **first goal** is you have to view each and every day as being *split into two parts*. Each day should be viewed as having both a *first part* and *a second part*. The first part is the morning and afternoon.

The second part is late afternoon and evening until it's time for bed. However, if you happen to have a different waking cycle due to working night shift or any other reason, it's your job to decide on how you're going to split your day up into the two parts.

The **second goal** that you have to hit every day is making sure that during the second part of your day, you intentionally perform the actions that will get you into the slight state of *negative energy balance* required in order for all weight and body fat loss to occur overnight while you sleep.

These actions consist of first reducing your caloric intake during this half of the day, consuming only one moderately sized highly nutritious meal consisting of lean protein and vegetables only. You must make sure that you're thoroughly educated on carbohydrates so that you know the difference between fibrous carbs and starchy carbs. *Fibrous carbs,* such as vegetables and fruits, should be the only carbohydrates you consume during the second part of your day as they are very low in calories, high in essential nutrients and do not stimulate fat storage.

Starchy carbohydrates are your breads, rice, potatoes, pastas, oats and other heavier carbohydrates. You must not eat these after about 2pm. By eating smaller portions, yet keeping the food of the highest nutritional quality, fresh vegetables, lean cuts of protein and a tiny amount of omega-3 fats, you will minimise the calories you consume, yet fully satisfy and provide all the essential nutrients for growth and repair as the result of your daily activities.

The order to eat specific types of foods over the course of your day:

You want to eat a high quality, moderate to large sized nutritious breakfast, a light lunch and a smaller evening meal. If you're experiencing true physical hunger between your meals that negatively impact your performance or mood, then you may snack on a high quality lean source of protein.

After your evening meal, you should not eat any more food unless it's a small portion of high quality lean protein in the form of a snack to feed your body of uncomfortable physical hunger. In addition if you enjoy eating starchy carbohydrates such as bread, rice, pasta, potatoes and cereals, then make the commitment to eat more of these during the morning, a little in the afternoon and none whatsoever during the evening.

By eating them *earlier* in your day, you will most likely put the nutrients contained in them to good use as fuel for all the tasks and activities you're faced with. However, later on you want to keep your body starchy carbohydrate-free so that any energy required for activity or bodily functions during the evening, particularly while you're sleeping, will be obtained from your body fat stores as there are no carbohydrate sugars in your system to draw upon.

Your muscles, cells and body systems grow and repair while you're asleep. However, they require energy to do this. If you do not eat any carbohydrates, your body will then shift on to using any of your stored body fat for energy to fuel the recovery processes instead, resulting in weight loss and burning off unwanted body fat. The right mind-set towards the size or quantity of your meals as well as the amount of starchy carbohydrates included over the course of your day, should be truly understood and adopted.

If you manage create a habit out of this way of approaching each and every one of your days, it will only be a matter of time before you will be naturally walking around at a lighter, leaner version of yourself for the rest of your life. Provided you stick to this habit religiously and do not revert back to your old ways. This is illustrated in Figure 6.

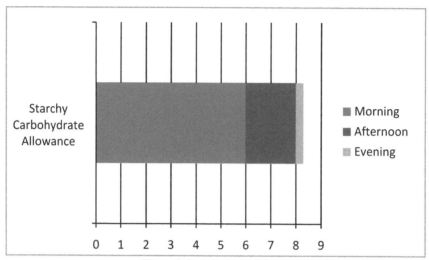

Figure 6: Carbohydrates Allowance

Following this one strategy will achieve significant results.

The most effective means of losing weight and body fat, even more than exercise is the application of The Pareto Principle (the 80/20 rule) as discussed earlier. 20% of the foods you eat will be responsible for 80% of your desired outcome, where 80% of the food you eat will lead to results of a more undesirable outcome.

Not only should this principle be applied to the quality of foods you eat, which would be lean proteins, lots of vegetables, some fruits and a little omega-3 healthy fats, but also the quantity of food you eat throughout your day. 80% of your food should be consumed during the first half of your day, during the morning and afternoon.

This ensures the food is used directly as quality fuel for you throughout your day, where as 20% of your food should be consumed during the second half of your day between your evening meal and bedtime. After your evening meal at around five or six in the evening, you should only eat if a high degree of uncomfortable physical hunger is experienced.

Your Nutrition– Diet Improvement Brainstorming Exercise

Every week, month, year, and over the course of your life as you strive to improve your physical, health and wellbeing you should always review and ask the question: "How can I improve my current eating routine?" You need to be aware of what you're eating and how to bring a greater scope of variety and quality to your meals. Don't try to be perfect because perfection does not exist. However always try to improve on your current habits and eating choices.

1. The first step to improving your current eating patterns, and therefore how your body appears in shape and size, is to grab a sheet of paper and a pen. Down the left hand side of your paper, number one to ten. Beside each number write down any of the foods you feel are not the most conductive towards weight and body fat loss. Write down all the foods you believe you can either eliminate from your diet or replace with healthier alternatives.

2. Next to this list of foods you wish to replace, write what you will replace them with: new fresh nutritious alternatives.

3. Now at the bottom of your sheet of paper, underneath your one to ten numbered brainstorming. Write a heading "Action Plan". Under this heading, on the left hand side of your paper, write the numbers one to five underneath each other. Alongside each number, write a new action you will implement to change what you eat each day. For example; no syrups in my Starbucks coffee. Or swap potatoes for extra vegetables in my evening meal. Buy fresh vegetables, prepare and cook them myself instead of buying ready-packaged vegetables from the supermarket and so on.

4. Put down your brainstorming piece of paper, go into the kitchen and rearrange your kitchen to reflect your new improvement-based choices. Or take action by writing a whole new, higher quality shopping list and then taking a trip to the supermarket for the week's supplies. Whatever positive action you can take to

improve your current eating patterns, will allow you to move forward and look and feel your very best. **Improvement should always be your focus.**

Part 2 – Your Activity

Once you have your diet firmly under control, assess your daily and weekly exercise patterns. In order for you to achieve maximum results in your body composition and overall health, choose a variety of exercises from those outlined earlier. Make full use of your exercise monthly calendar and diary.

Part 3 – Your Positive Life habits

Choose habits that are most relevant and practical to your own current life situation. Start with just one or two different activities or ways of approaching your day, then once these have been established through repetition over a period of a few weeks, incorporate another empowering habit and put them into continual action until they become second nature. The more empowering habits you have working for you, the sooner and greater the results in your physique and health.

Part 4 – Your Strategies

All it could take is one well-placed strategy to turn one of your problems or weaknesses into a powerful force. Look through the chapter on strategies and decide what will work best for you. Whether it's hiring a personal trainer to preparing your own lunches for work, start with just one strategy and put it into action. Once this strategy is working for you, consider implementing additional strategies.

Part 5 – Your Supplements

Once you have spent the time required to get your diet, activity levels, habits and strategies into your everyday life, you can further accelerate your progress by including any of the essential supplements into your daily routine.

Part 6 – Put your Mind-set to Work for You

After thoroughly reading, making your best efforts to relate to and understand the principles explained on the chapter on mind-set you now need to have complete faith and belief in these new ways of thinking and acting. At first, they may seem very vague or unrealistic to you. However by just putting your faith in them and taking actions you will begin to gain new levels of understanding and you will notice how these mind-set principles actually have a powerful effect on the outcome of your efforts.

Summary Diagram

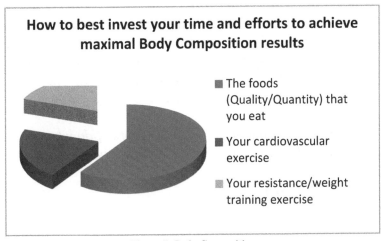

Figure 7: Body Composition

- Conclusion -

Now that you have all the practical guidelines you need to follow daily, and have created your own individual plan of action, all that is required from you now is **continual, ongoing action.** With self-analysis and reflection you have the tools to make slight adjustments along the way.

Embrace change, welcome growth. Success comes to all of us if we continually put our knowledge into action. Remember, we all have the same twenty-four hours in each day **but the difference in the quality of results is in the quality of the action we take.**

"Success is the progressive realization of a worthy ideal."
— **Earl Nightingale**

Everything Counts

The 'Everything-Counts' rule says that *everything you do or do not do each day either helps, or hinders your results.* Go to the gym, help yourself; don't go to the gym, hinder yourself. Nothing is neutral, every little thing or event affects the result. Therefore find the best way to combine my teachings to the best possible effect.

> *"Self-discipline is the ability to make yourself do what you should do, when you should do it, whether you feel like it or not."*
> — **Elbert Hubbard**

No Shortcuts

You won't get out, if you don't put in. There are no shortcuts to being the 'new you' you desire. The results, or lack of results that you ultimately achieve, will come in direct proportion to the energy, focus and effort you invest. There are many ways you can increase your effectiveness, but there are no shortcuts, no quick-fixes and no instant gratifications. Always remember: the greater effort, and time you invest, the sweeter the victory.

> *"Knowing is not enough, we must apply. Willing is not enough, we must do."*
> **– Bruce Lee**

Persist Until You Succeed

The most common reason people fail is they don't fight hard or long enough; they want the quick fixes when really they need to find the resolve and focus for the long-haul. Nothing is achieved overnight. Persistence is the only way forward. Two steps forward, one back, is the natural rhythm of life: accept that. It is all part of the process. But if you persist, you will achieve, as long as you keep taking small steps.

Rarely do we find a finer example of persistence than Abraham Lincoln. Take a look at some of the events that occurred over the period of Lincoln's life as he continued to work towards achieving his goals and becoming successful. Let this be your inspiration.

1. His mother dies.
2. His sister dies.
3. His business fails.
4. He runs for the State Legislature and loses. In the same year he also loses his job then applies to get into Law School and is rejected.
5. He then borrows money from a friend to begin a second business, which fails and leaves him bankrupt. It takes him seventeen years to pay off this debt.
6. He runs for the State Legislature again, this time he wins.

7. This year, things finally begin to look better for him as he is engaged and soon to be married. Unfortunately, his fiancée dies and he is left heartbroken.
8. He then has a complete nervous breakdown which leaves him in bed for six months.
9. He seeks to become speaker of the State Legislature. He is defeated.
10. He seeks to become Elector. He is defeated.
11. He marries another woman and they have had four boys together. Only one of them lives to maturity.
12. He then runs for Senate of the United States. He loses.
13. He runs for Congress and loses.
14. He runs for Congress again, this time he wins. He then goes to Washington and does well.
15. He runs for re-election for Congress. He loses.
16. He runs for the Senate of the United States again. He loses.
17. He seeks the job as a land officer in his home state. He is rejected.
18. He runs for the Vice President of the United States, he loses.
19. He runs for the Senate of the United States again. He loses, again.
20. **He is elected as the President of the United States of America.**

As you can see, despite all of his setbacks, Lincoln never lost sight of the belief that he could make a positive difference in the world. He maintained his confidence in his abilities and persevered through every obstacle and setback, learning from each experience and getting himself right back on track. As you look at your own life, is there a noble, audacious aim that you have given up on after multiple set-backs? Looking at the time-line of Abraham Lincoln's life, when would you have given up? Failure, is only a signal to try again more intelligently. Learn the lessons contained in each one of your failures and then continue to move ahead, until you *eventually* succeed.

"Failure is simply the opportunity to begin again, this time more intelligently."
– Henry Ford

Not So Serious

You should never get to the point where you get too carried away with your physique and health goals that you begin to neglect other areas of your life. Life is to be lived fully, so make an effort to celebrate your progress and improvements along the way.

Being able to relax, every now and again, such as at the weekends, will help you to stay on the right course and maintain that all essential balance in life. As long as around 80% of your actions and efforts are positive and moving you in the direction of your goals, allow yourself to be human and let your hair down for around 20% or less of the time.

Stopping for short breaks to celebrate your progress and efforts every now and again, as well as encouraging and cheering on your friends, family members or spouse's progress are all very important. If you have been entrusted with other people's commitments to improving their looks and health, then make sure that you take on the part of an uplifting, positive force by giving them genuine recognition and praise where deserved.

Celebrate their progress. Consider giving them a shopping voucher to their favourite shop; take them out for a meal, book a weekend away. By contributing to other people in your life as a way of acknowledging their efforts and commitments, you will become a dominant positive force in their lives

Never Look Back

After reading this book, learning and applying the key principles to your life and developing yourself to become the best you can be, you need to understand the one principle that it all comes down to in the end. And that is: **it never ends.**

You will have to make real and sustainable changes to your lifestyle... and that means *forever*. You will exercise, buy foods, cook foods, sleep, breathe and live out the philosophy given to you in this book. When you begin to change, everything in your world will change and improve around you as a by-product. You are the trigger, nobody else can do your push ups for you. But once you stay committed to your new ways, your new ways will then stay loyal and committed to you.

"The best way to predict the future is to invent it."
– Alan Kay

Final Words

I truly believe deep down, that it is not possible for anybody to feel at their best if they are not engaged in actions every single day that positively contribute to the journey of their own personal growth and development. Unfulfilled potential can lead only to dissatisfaction.

Practice, master and transform.

I greatly appreciate you all for taking the time to read this book. You are the only person who is responsible for your own fate – so no more excuses, only continual, everyday ongoing positive action. Never stop improving and striving to be better today than you were yesterday. And just imagine what you'll be tomorrow.

"Man who waits for roast duck to fly into mouth must wait very, very long time."
– Chinese Proverb

Your personal Blueprint: Create your plan/ Do it NOW.

Below, is a chart that takes into account the **key result areas** that determine how you will look physically and how you will feel in terms of your energy, vitality and health. As you begin to make many new positive changes in your life in each of the following areas, forging out new habits to replace your current ways of doing things, check off the chart list one by one until you have mastered your health in each and every area.

Action	Implemented ☑	Mastered / Made habit in my life ☑
Applied Nutrition Principles	☐	☐
Planned and applied exercise routine on calendar	☐	☐
Included supplements	☐	☐
Applied positive habit 1:	☐	☐
Applied positive habit 2:	☐	☐
Applied positive habit 3:	☐	☐
Applied positive habit 4:	☐	☐
Applied positive habit 5:	☐	☐
Applied Strategy 1:	☐	☐
Applied Strategy 2:	☐	☐
Applied Strategy 3:	☐	☐
Applied Strategy 4:	☐	☐
Applied Strategy 5:	☐	☐

"Go for it now, the future is promised to no one."
– Dr. Wayne Dyer